Techniques in Percutaneous Renal Stone Surgery

Subodh R. Shivde
Editor

Techniques in Percutaneous Renal Stone Surgery

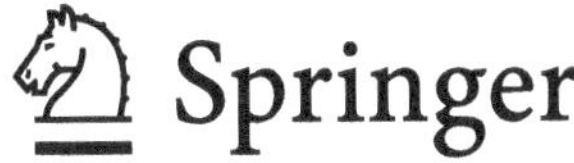

Springer

Editor
Subodh R. Shivde
Urosurgery and Transplant Services
Deenanath Mangeshkar Hospital and Resear
Pune, Maharashtra, India

ISBN 978-981-19-9420-3 ISBN 978-981-19-9418-0 (eBook)
https://doi.org/10.1007/978-981-19-9418-0

This Springer imprint is published by the registered company Springer Nature Singapore Pte Ltd.
The registered company address is: 152 Beach Road, #21-01/04 Gateway East, Singapore 189721, Singapore

This practical book on Percutaneous Renal Surgery for Renal Stone is dedicated to my teachers ***Dr. Madhumalti Herlekar, Dr. Dev S Pardanani, Dr. Sulbha Punekar, Mr. Graham Watson****,* ***my students, my patients*** *and last but not least to my beloved wife* ***Dr. Bhagyashree*** *and my son* ***Sujoy*** *whose constant support and encouragement led me to persevere and finish the project.*

Preface

Why do we need a new book on Percutaneous Renal Surgery? As a matter of fact, why do we need any information in this day and age of the internet in a book form when all we have to do is get online? Books serve as a resource where experts have added their valuable clinical experience to the currently available information and knowledge base.

We endeavour to gather the pearls of wisdom from clinical experts in a logically linear manner to help newcomers—students and young urology practitioners approach the common and not-so-common scenarios in Percutaneous Renal Surgery.

We try to work up a typical and not-so-typical 'PCNL patient' as we would do in our day-to-day practice. The book is not a substitute for the existing textbooks and monograms on Percutaneous Renal Surgery but would serve as a good practical handbook for ready reference with many practical add-ons as workup for a typical patient, tips and tricks, troubleshooting and some not so commonly thought of practices such as exit strategies. The book also touches upon newer methods adopted by urologists such as supine PCNL and miniaturization of the conventional instruments to 'The Mini' and 'The Micro' PCNL systems. The most dreaded part of the Percutaneous Renal Surgery is the access difficulty and the complications which ensue, and this has been adequately elaborated in the two chapters devoted to it.

No practical book on operating surgery would be complete without elaborating on the training and teaching aspect for this surgery, and we have tried to gather the currently available know-how in the chapter 'Training in PCNL'.

The current monogram ends with a biochemical workup of the stones and the practically useful tests which help patient counselling.

The team of authors have tried to look into the future of Percutaneous Renal Surgery with the chapter 'Future of Percutaneous Renal Surgery' entering the new era of science and technology to help both the modern surgeon and patients.

Pune, Maharashtra, India — Subodh R. Shivde

Contents

Contributors

Amruta Bedekar, MD, FRCA Deenanath Mangeshkar Hospital and Research Centre, Pune, India

Jaspreet Singh Chabra, MS, DNB (Uro) Muljibhai Patel Urological Hospital, Nadiad, Gujarat, India

Gajanan Chaudhary, MS (Gen Surgery) Department of Urology, Deenanath Mangeshkar Hospital and Research Centre, Pune, Maharashtra, India

Jaydeep Date, MS, MCh Deenanath Mangeshkar Hospital, Pune, India

Mahesh R. Desai, MS, FRCS Muljibhai Patel Urological Hospital, Nadiad, Gujarat, India

Sanjay Deshpande, MS, FRCS Solapur, Maharashtra, India

Arvind P. Ganpule, MS, DNB Muljibhai Patel Urological Hospital, Nadiad, Gujarat, India

Rakesh Jamkhandikar, MD, FRCR, M Med (Singapore) North Cumbria Integrated Care NHS Trust UK, Carlisle, UK

Rajesh Kukreja, MS, DNB (Urology) Urocare Hospital, Indore, India

Chetan Kulkarni, MS, DNB Kolhapur, Maharashtra, India

Pankaj N. Maheshwari, MS, MCh Fortis Hospital, Mumbai, India

Sanjeev Mehta, MD Uro Lab, Ahmedabad, India

V. Mohankumar, MS, DNB (Urosurgery) Department of Urology, Muljibhai Patel Urological Hospital, Nadiad, Gujarat, India

Ashish V. Rawandale-Patil, MS, MCh Institute of Urology Dhule, Dhule, Maharashtra, India

Lokesh Patni, MS, DNB Institute of Urology Dhule, Dhule, Maharashtra, India

Abhay Rane, OBE, FRCS (Urol) East Surrey Hospital, Redhill, UK

Ravindra Sabnis, MCH (urology) Department of Urology, Muljibhai Patel Urological Hospital (MPUH), Nadiad, Gujarat, India

S. Segaran, MS, FRCS Damansara Specialist Hospital 2, Kuala Lumpur, Malaysia

Lalit Shah, MS, MCh Raipur, India

Bhagyashree Shivde, MD, FRCA, DA (London) Deenanath Mangeshkar Hospital and Research Centre, Pune, India

Subodh R. Shivde, MCh FRCS(Uro)FEBU Department of Urology, Deenanath Mangeshkar Hospital and Research Centre, Pune, Maharashtra, India

Department of Urology Transplant and Robotics, Deenanath Mangeshkar Hospital, Pune, India

Abhishek Singh, MCH (urology) Department of Urology, MPUH, Nadiad, India

Rohan Valsangkar, MS, MCh Deenanath Mangeshkar Hospital, Pune, India

Anatomy for Percutaneous Renal Surgery and Access to Pelvicalyceal System

1

Gajanan Chaudhary and Subodh R. Shivde

1.1 Introduction

Kidneys are bean-shaped paired structures situated in the retroperitoneum. They are situated over the psoas muscles along the axis of the muscle thereby causing them to be at an angle of about 30°–50° to the coronal plane and are typically placed so that their hila containing the vessels are placed medially and facing anteriorly. Typically the broader upper poles are more medially placed and the convex outer borders are more posterior [1] (Fig. 1.1).

G. Chaudhary · S. R. Shivde (✉)
Department of Urology, Deenanath Mangeshkar Hospital and Research Centre, Pune, Maharashtra, India

S. R. Shivde (ed.), *Techniques in Percutaneous Renal Stone Surgery*, https://doi.org/10.1007/978-981-19-9418-0_1

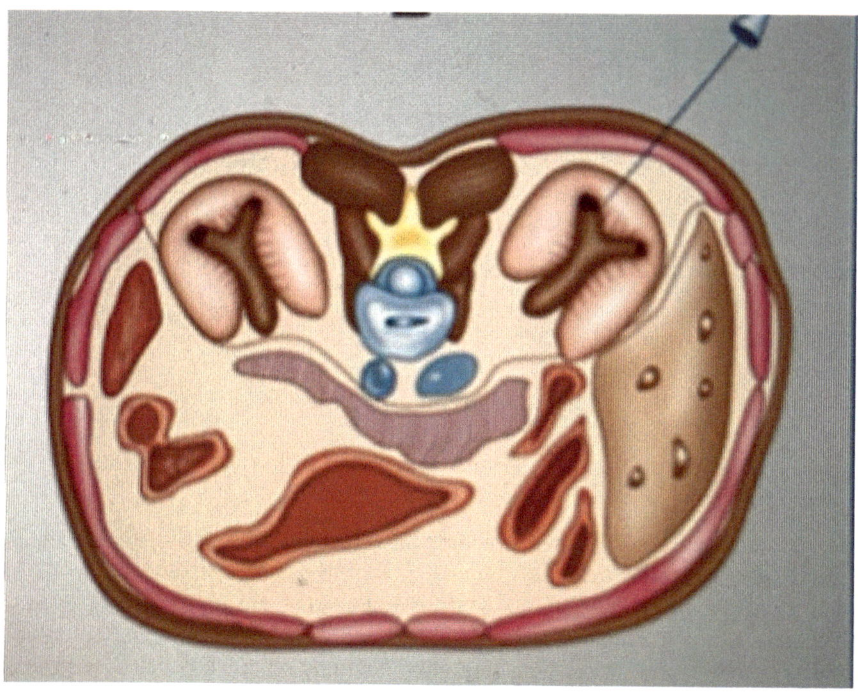

Fig. 1.1 Schematic representation of orientation of kidneys in prone position and their relation to other structures. (Please note the direct entry of correctly placed needle in posterior calyx of the right kidney)

1.2 Kidney Coverings and Relations of Other Organs

Each kidney has a true renal capsule blended tightly with the parenchyma and a loose layer of fibrofatty tissue consisting of loose areolar tissue which divides the spaces around the kidney into pararenal space, medial hilar space consisting of entry and exit of renal hilar vessels and the renal pelvis. Superiorly the fascia covers the suprarenal glands and is in close contact with the inner surface of the diaphragm.

The lateral relations of the right kidney from the superior to the inferior pole are the liver and ascending colon duodenum medial and anteriorly. On the left side, the kidney has spleen superiorly and the descending colon anteriorly and laterally. The tail of the pancreas is in medial relation to the hilum of the left kidney (Fig. 1.2).

In a study by Sengupta et al. it was proved that patient position, prone or supine had no change in orientation of the kidneys [2]. The orientation of kidneys from midsagittal plane changed from 56.6° to 61.6°. The orientation of calyces, both anterior and posterior showed no clinically significant change when studied on CT IVU studies taking 5 mm cuts [3].

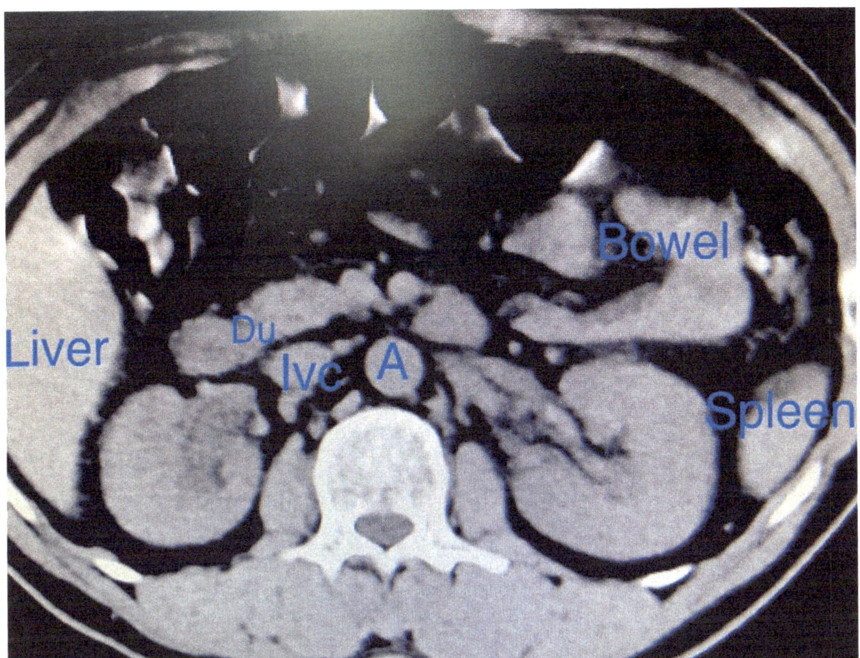

Fig. 1.2 CT picture showing the cross-sectional anatomy of relations of kidneys (*Du* duodenum, *IVC* inferior vena cava, *A* aorta)

1.3 Intrarenal Vessels [3]

1.3.1 Renal Artery

The main renal artery arising from the aorta at the level of L1 vertebra divides into anterior and posterior branches. The posterior branch is retro pelvic, and it supplies the segment posteriorly without further branching (Fig. 1.3).

The anterior branch of the renal artery in the hilum divides into segmental branches (apical, upper middle and lower divisions). Each further divides into interlobar and then interlobular (infundibular) branches. These are close to the infundibulum and are in direct contact with the calyces. Further division of these give rise to arcuate arteries which enter pyramid and then subdivide to form the afferent arteriole of glomerulus.

The infundibula are in close relation to arteries and any puncture through this region has risks of bleeding significantly. The relative risk of injury to infundibular vessels in upper pole, middle pole and lower pole is 57%, 23% and 13% respectively. This confirms the safety of lower polar puncture.

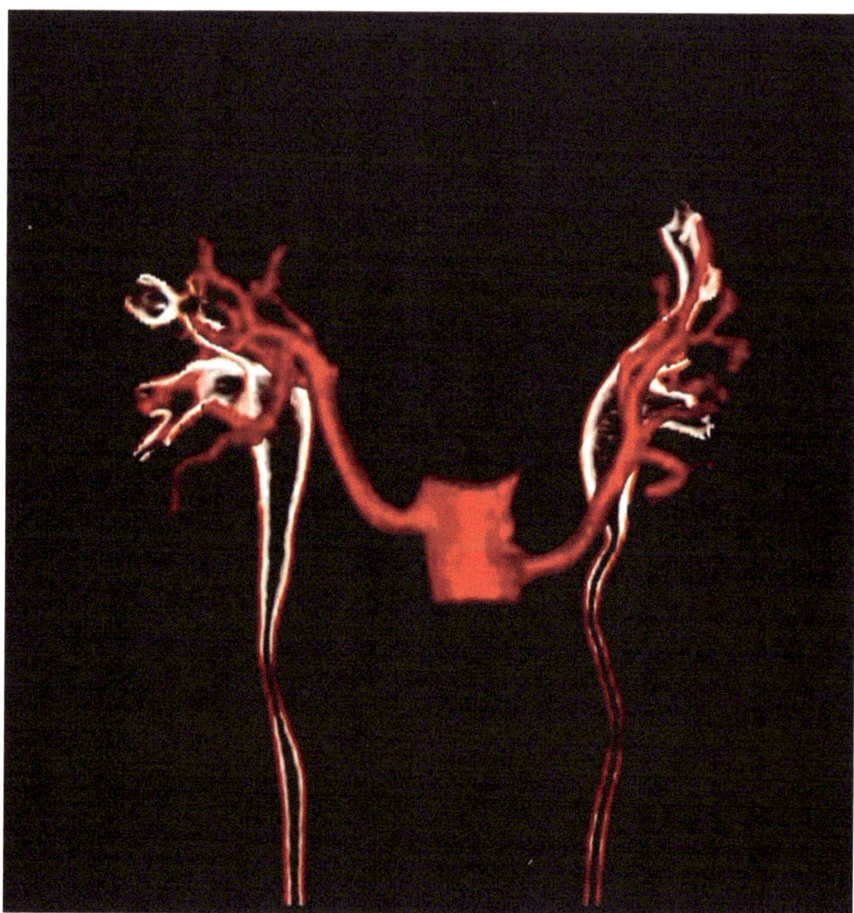

Fig. 1.3 CT angio reconstruction showing the two renal arteries arising at the level of vertebra (L1) branching into the anterior and posterior divisions with further subdivisions. Please note the close relationship to the normal pelvicalyceal system

There is a plane of relatively avascular field between the branching network of anterior and posterior divisions of renal artery popularly known as Brodel's avascular plane. The prone position of the patient allows going through this to enter renal parenchyma with minimal vascular injury (Fig. 1.4).

1.3.2 Renal Vein

The intrarenal veins do not have a segmental or lobar pattern unlike arterial system. They are seen arranged as arcades and freely intercommunicate. A variable number of 2–4 trunks are seen in varying proportions. As a result of the free communication,

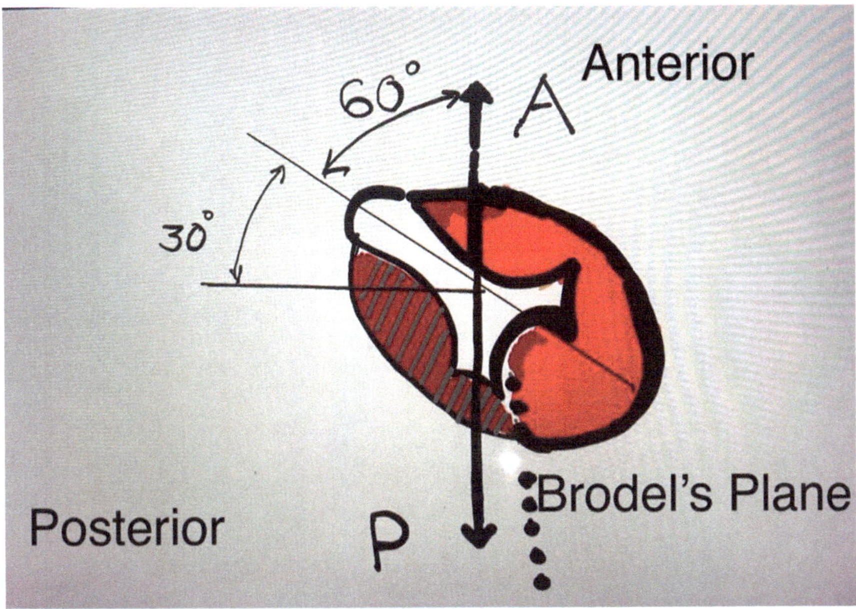

Fig. 1.4 Division of anterior and posterior branches of renal artery and areas supplied in kidney with depiction of Brodel's plane

the effects of injury to veins such as ischaemic events are not very harmful to the renal parenchyma (Fig. 1.5).

1.3.3 Pelvicalyceal System

The minor calyces which are generally present in 5–14 numbers (mean of 8) will be seen adjacent to renal pyramid thus draining it. Minor calyces are single or compound draining 2–3 papillae. Compound calyces are generally present near poles. The minor calyces drain straight into the infundibulum or join to form major calyces. Finally, the infundibula drain into the pelvis (Fig. 1.6).

The posterior calyces are typically rotated 30° and hence allow puncture directly in percutaneous renal surgery in prone position. The anatomy in cases of congenital anomalies such as horse shoe or renal ectopia follows a different pattern and would need detailed study of radiological images.

The patterns of pelvicalyceal system are complex and highly variable even between right and left sides in the same patient. Numerous endocast studies and cadaveric dissection studies with anatomical correlation have proved that these patterns have such a variability that no general scheme can be found for percutaneous surgery. The punctures should be performed through papilla of the calyx which is the least traumatic possibly injuring only the small marginal vessel and or small

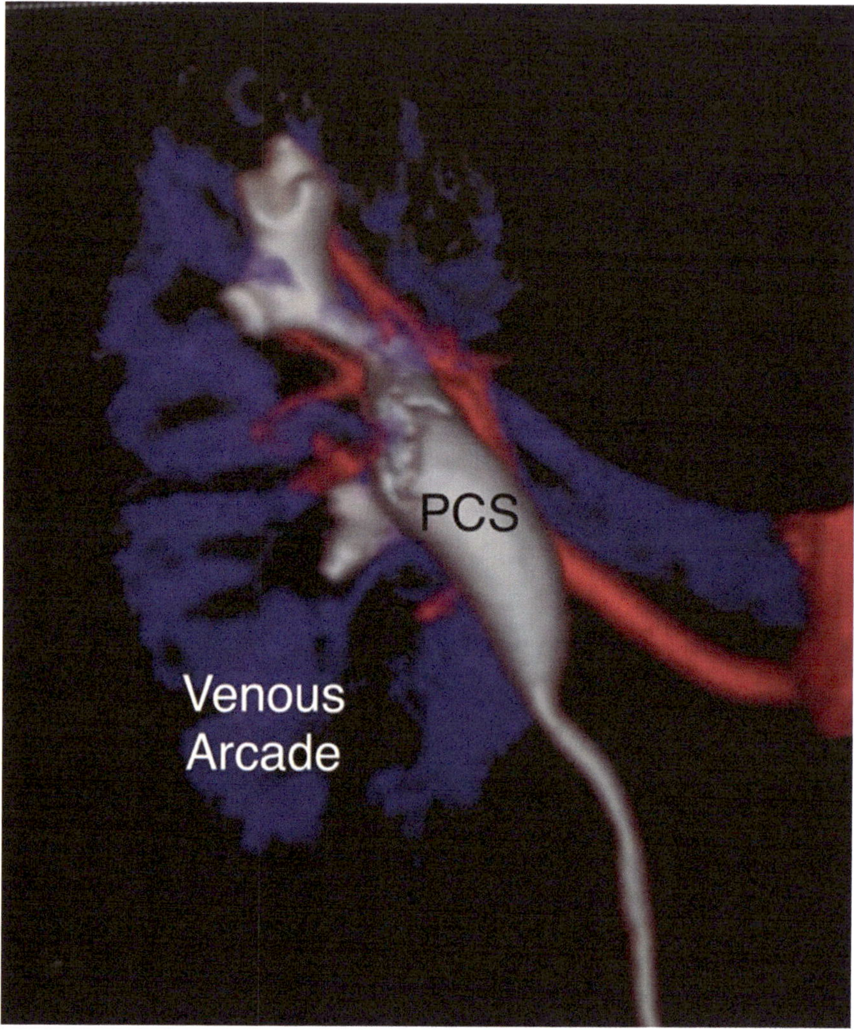

Fig. 1.5 CT reconstruction of left kidney showing venous arcade and drainage in two main trunks then merging in left renal vein. Please note the close relation to PCS (pelvicalyceal system)

venules. The puncture should never be done through the fornix as it is liable to damage segmental vessel. Injury to the posterior segmental branch may lead to major haemorrhage and can result in significant loss of parenchyma [4].

Puncture should never be performed through renal pelvis as the instruments would get dislodged easily and maintaining a tract will not be possible. It is associated with a very high complication rate [5].

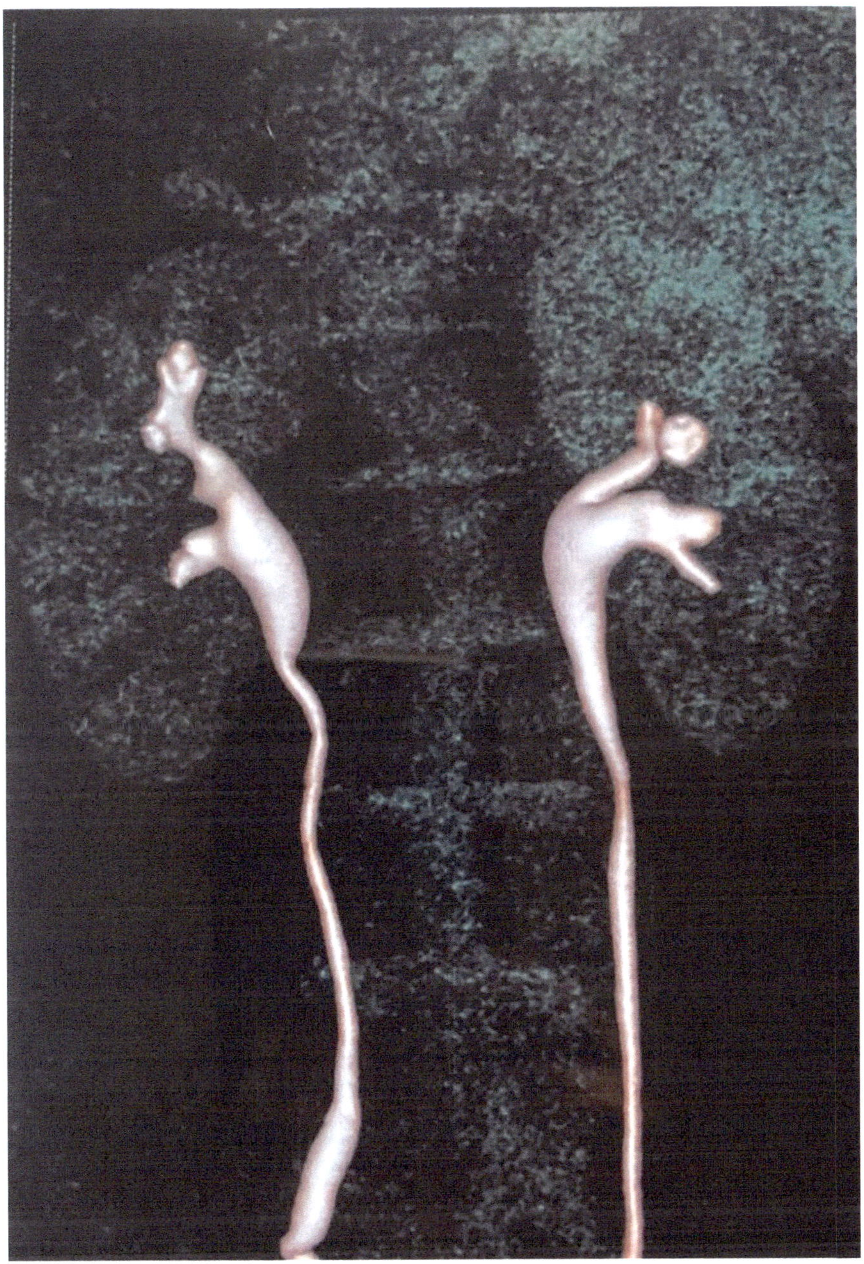

Fig. 1.6 CT reconstruction showing pelvicalyceal system

References

1. Sampaio FJ, et al. Morphometry of the kidney. Applied study in urology and imaging. J D'urol. 1989;95(2):77–80.
2. Sengupta S, Donnellan S, Vincent JM, Webb DR. CT analysis of caliceal anatomy in the supine and prone positions. J Endourol. 2000;14(7):555–7.
3. Sampaio FJ, Aragao AH. Anatomical relationship between the intrarenal arteries and the kidney collecting system. J Urol. 1990;143(4):679–81.
4. Sampaio FJB, Mandarim-De-Lacerda CA. Anatomic classification of the kidney collecting system for endourologic procedures. J Endourol. 1988;2:247–51. https://doi.org/10.1089/end.1988.2.247.
5. Smith's Textbook of Endourology—Arthur D. Smith—Google Books. https://books.google.co.in/books?hl=en&lr=&id=Wo8cgdAsL-EC&oi=fnd&pg=PA1&dq=Smith%27s+textbook+of+Endourology&ots=4979fdxrmC&sig=z5svgt0ZTmLc5kVwlvG7FOSxFRo&redir_esc=y#v=onepage&q=Smith's%20textbook%20of%20Endourology&f=false. Accessed 17 Jul 2022.

Imaging for Percutaneous Renal Surgery

2

Subodh R. Shivde and Rakesh Jamkhandikar

2.1 Introduction and Surgical Anatomy

Traditionally access to the kidney has been evolving since Goodwin described the first renal percutaneous procedure [1]. Since then, a number of radiological techniques have been employed to gain access to the renal pelvicalyceal system and here is the overview.

2.2 Relevant Surgical Anatomy

Kidneys are retroperitoneal organs which are surrounded by many organs and major vessels. Access to the kidney, therefore, is a very specialised act and needs a very careful understanding of the surgical anatomy of structures and also the physics of all instruments.

The kidneys are highly mobile organs typically moving in the craniocaudal line by 3–5 cm. Both kidneys are oriented ventromedially and are in relation to L1 lumbar vertebra. The right kidney is in close relationship to the liver anteriorly and superiorly, duodenum and vena cava anteriorly and medially and colon anteriorly. The left kidney with spleen laterally and the aorta and tail of the pancreas medially and anteriorly, the colon anteriorly.

The frontal plane of the kidneys is 30° posterior to the coronal plane of the body.

S. R. Shivde
Department of Urology, Deenanath Mangeshkar Hospital and Research Centre, Pune, Maharashtra, India

R. Jamkhandikar (✉)
North Cumbria Integrated Care NHS Trust UK, Carlisle, UK

S. R. Shivde (ed.), *Techniques in Percutaneous Renal Stone Surgery*, https://doi.org/10.1007/978-981-19-9418-0_2

The calyceal anatomy varies in the right and left kidneys. The posterior calyces are positioned 20° posteriorly to the frontal plane in most right kidneys and 70° posterior to the frontal plane in majority of left kidneys.

2.3 Percutaneous Renal Access Without Image Guidance

2.3.1 Indications

1. Emergent situations needing drainage of hydronephrotic dilated system.
2. Situations where normal access such as insertion of ureteric catheter into the pelvicalyceal system has failed (not able to see or enter the ureteric opening due to visualisation problems, bleeding bladder mucosa, severely trabeculated bladder).

2.4 The Technique

The preoperative counselling consists of information about the approach and possible higher complication rates in view of difficult access. The need for multiple needle punctures is explained. All preoperative checks such as urine tests and preoperative coagulation profile and antibiotic prophylaxis are followed as per standard PCNL procedure.

The lumbar notch is identified which has the 12th rib and latissimus dorsi as the superior margin, the medial margin consisting of quadratus lumborum and sacrospinalis muscles, and the lateral border formed by external oblique and transversus abdominis muscles. The needle entry starts after infiltration of local anaesthetic just below the 12th rib. The needle choice is an 18 G needle with stilette which can be passed without much tissue resistance. The needle is pushed about 4–5 cm in the cephalic direction. The needle moves up and down with respiration when in renal cortex. The position is confirmed by aspiration with a 2 cc syringe which draws clear fluid, i.e. urine. The advantage of the 18 G needle is that a 0.035 guide wire can be passed into the collecting system which then takes the shape of the system allowing us to know the right placement. The correct access can also be confirmed by injection small amount of diluted contrast material. In difficult cases, a long 22 G spinal puncture needle can be used and then position can be confirmed by injecting a contrast medium. This needle has the advantage that the puncture leads to very little vascular injury and a negligible amount of trauma to surrounding structures if access is through some other surrounding structures.

The current role of this technique should only be reserved for emergency situations where imaging is not available and is discouraged due to the high complication rate which includes bleeding and blind entry into the pelvicalyceal system [2].

2.4.1 Complications

1. Bleeding
2. Infections and septic events
3. Pleural punctures in cases of supracostal punctures leading to pneumothorax

2.5 Conventional Imaging Using Image Intensifier (II)

After the first description of percutaneous access to kidney by Goodwin in 1955, Fernstorm and Johansson described their first experience of three patients of percutaneous removal of kidney stones using image guidance [3]. While this involved a slow dilation of tract over 7 days, Alken showed and pioneered a technique of gradual one step dilation using specialised polyethylene tubes and then metal dilators which telescope in over the guide rod which is placed over the wire. The entire procedure is done using image guidance with image intensifier [4]. Arthur Smith and group eventually confirmed the safety of rapid dilation without any adverse effects to popularise the currently practiced method [5].

Fluoroscopy using image intensifier uses 2D imaging for the entire sequence of percutaneous surgery which includes access to the pelvicalyceal system, insertion of guide wire, dilatation of the tract and then insertion of Amplatz sheath. The procedure utilises the endoscopic view of the nephroscope and the images from the II to monitor the progress of the procedure and monitor the clearance of stones and look for the residual stones. The disadvantage if II is that it does not localise or image the solid organs surrounding the kidney. It will allow screening in a limited manner to see for some inadvertent complications such as the development of pneumothorax and sometimes the presence of retro renal colon.

2.5.1 The Technique [6]

A rigid cystoscopy is performed under suitable anaesthesia, and a ureteric catheter is inserted in the ureter gaining access to the desired pelvicalyceal system. We hereby describe the commonly performed prone approach with two techniques, namely the triangulation technique and the Bulls eye method.

There are 5 points which need to be remembered before any puncture method is adopted in PCNL

1. Access through posterolateral approach
2. Through the renal parenchyma
3. Towards the centre of the calyx posterolaterally
4. Towards the centre of the renal pelvis
5. Remember the Brodel's avascular plain with minimum vasculature

A strict adherence to the above would result in safe punctures without serious complications.

2.6 The Triangulation Technique

With the patient in the prone position, all pressure parts/points padded and special care to be taken in the patients intubated and under suitable antibiotic cover. A diluted contrast with a coloured fluid such as methylene blue is then injected via the adapter into the ureteric catheter and one of the following methods or combination is adopted.

This involves the geometric principles using the BI PLANAR fluoroscopy. The A-P view is parallel to the axis of puncture and monitors the mediolateral (LEFT to RIGHT) adjustments.

In the oblique view, the II is tilted 30° to the head end or foot end giving an idea about the cephalad–caudal movements. The operator should only adjust either mediolateral or cephalocaudal needle placement at one go. The anaesthetist is advised to hold the respiration in full expiration so that the target calyx is NOT a moving target.

In the A-P screening mode, a skin puncture is made so as to advance the puncture needle with stilette at an angle of about 30° to the back aiming at the desired calyx. A tissue resistance is met when needle meets the cortex of the kidney when some gentle pushing leads to movement of the contrast filled pelvicalyceal system. A give way is felt when the tip enters the system. Upon changing the C arm axis to 30°, the cephalocaudal orientation is checked (Fig. 2.1).

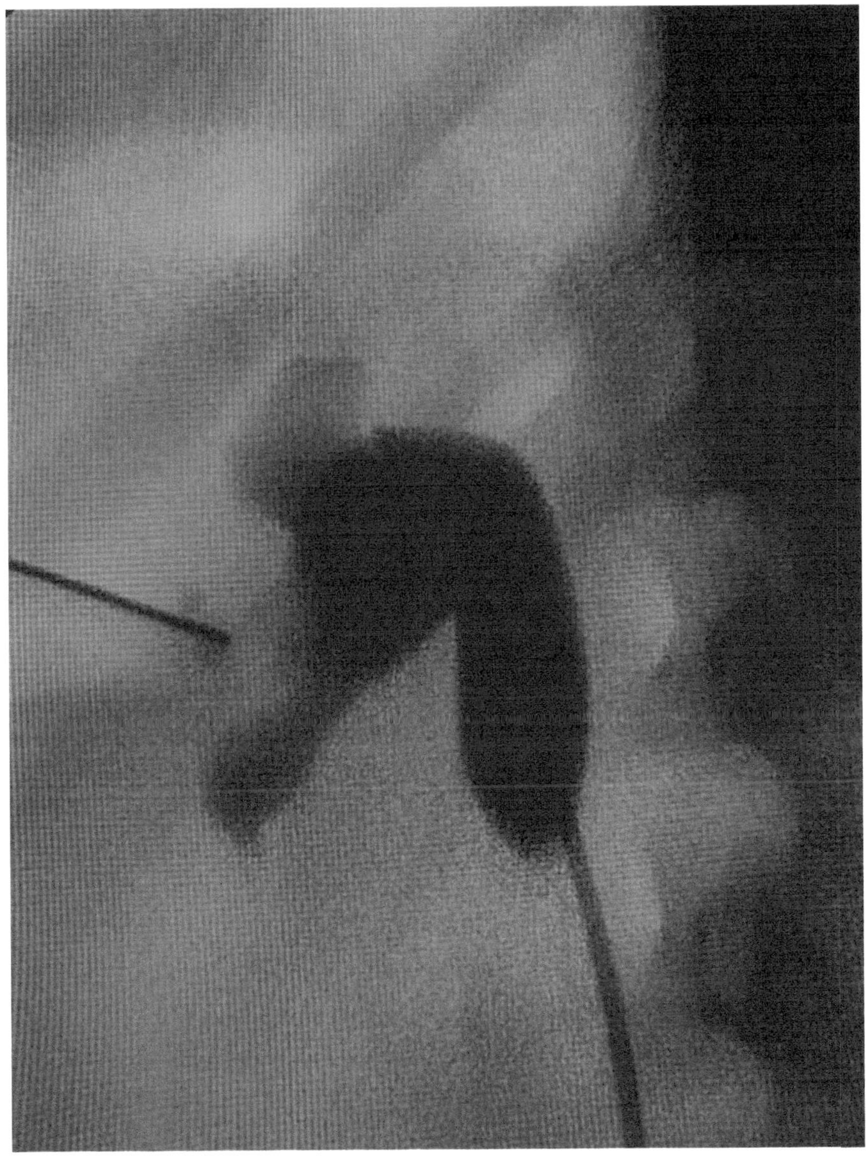

Fig. 2.1 The puncture needle is seen entering the less opacified posterior calyx by triangulation technique. (Also ref. to chapter Tips and Tricks)

2.7 Practical Tips

On AP screening and subsequent 30° tilt if the needle doesn't align with the target and is seen MEDIAL to it then consider it to be in SUPERFICIAL plane and then withdraw the needle out of the cortex and move again in a plane that is DEEPER. Similarly if the combined screening reveals the needle tip to be LATERAL to the entry point, then withdraw the needle and advance again in the SUPERFICIAL plane. The correct placement only conformed when there is free fluid seen oozing out from the needle and only then try and put in a soft flexible end glide wire to guide the surgery forward. DO NOT INSERT A GUIDE WIRE if the returning fluid is red suggesting inadvertent entry through a vessel. It's best to stop and start with a new puncture.

2.8 The Bulls Eye Technique

The target, i.e. the desired calyx and renal pelvis are in line of the puncture needle with the C arm rotated 30° so as to align the needle tip, the hub of the needle and the calyx are in the same plane so that the appearance is that of Bulls eye. In effect the

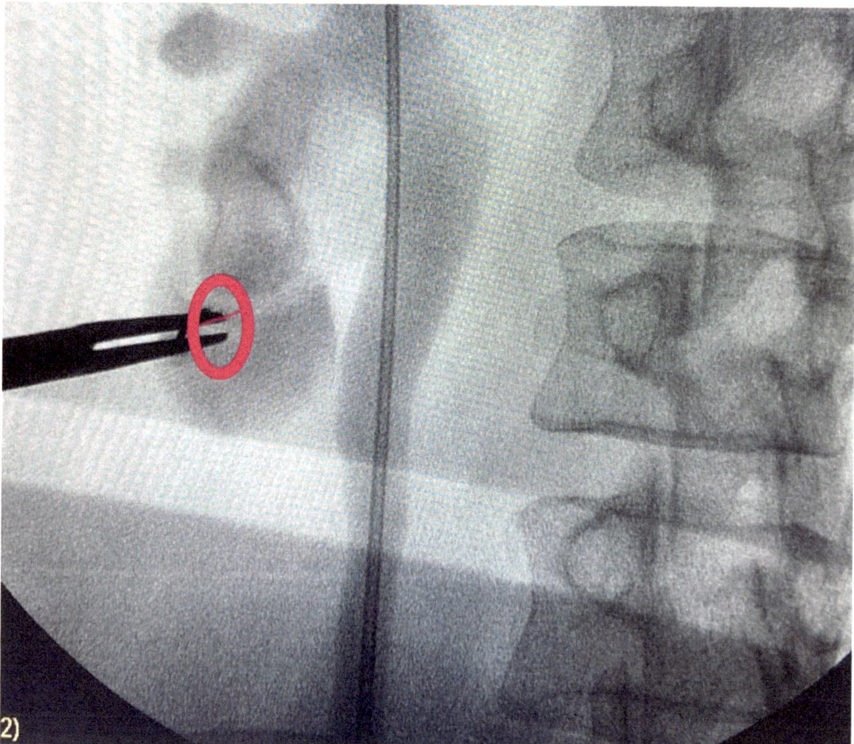

Fig. 2.2 Showing the 'end on' picture needle hub and calyx in one area (note the needle held by needle holder to avoid radiation exposure)

surgeon is looking down in the calyx (Fig. 2.2). The in-depth advancements are done with anteroposterior movement being monitored by constant screening. The entry is checked by withdrawing the stilette and checking aspiration of urine mixed with contrast by syringe.

2.9 Other Techniques

Some other surgeons have modified above-mentioned methods with variable combinations. Mues et al. [7] modified the above technique considering the plane of coincidence of C arm and the plane of needle entry showing a good reproducibility between different members of the team in 28 cases.

Miller et al. reviewed literature over 20 years relating to various techniques for obtaining access to pelvicalyceal system and concluded the established fact that a detailed anatomy of kidney and the knowledge of vascular system in relation to pelvicalyceal system was necessary for the puncturing of the system. A trend world over is to get help from radiology colleague to establish a tract before the percutaneous surgery [6]. In the eastern subcontinent however the urologists prefer to do their own tract by one of the convenient methods.

2.10 Multiple Punctures and Different Access Modifications

In cases where the stone burden is large as indicated by radiology workup preoperatively it would be prudent to plan punctures at suitable points of entry. While most stone bulk can be cleared with one puncture, additional punctures are made after parking the first wire in the initial puncture. Care should be taken to do these additional punctures before dilation of the tract to prevent contrast extravasation causing difficulties in visualising the optimum points of puncture. Multiple tracts made to clear large stone burden has definitely shown to improve stone free rates without additional morbidity [8].

2.11 Radiation Safety and Precautions

Component positioning uses the C arm in such a way that the II is above the patient and the tube is shielded by the table, thereby minimising the direct scatter. Doubling the distance from the source reduces the X-ray exposure to one fourth and tripling to one nineth, thus improving the safety. It is mandatory to wear appropriate safety shields in operating rooms and also use TLD badges to monitor exposure of theatre personnel.

Digital imaging and newer image storage facilities allow use of low doses of radiation using ALARA principle and keep the operating theatre team safe.

Use of ultrasound allows the surgeon to minimise radiation and also have better visualisation of vascular structures when using the B mode.

2.12 Intraoperative Ultrasonography and Obtaining the Access

2.12.1 Equipment

A convex probe of 3.5–5 MHz would be needed. An optimum combination would be a needle guide for fixing the needle and getting an electronic guide or trajectory to precisely localise the target calyx. A specially made puncture needle called Echo Tip Needle by Cook® which is scored so as to show a reflection as the tip enters the desired site. We however prefer to use 18 G needle with stilette which allows a passage of 0.035 inch or 0.038 inch flexible Terumo™ type wire.

2.13 The Ultrasound Guided Access

The procedure begins after positioning the patient prone. Some units prefer to use bolsters under the chest at the level of lower part of thoracic cage and at the level of pelvis in order to let the bowel fall down, thereby protecting them and preventing injury. We however do not use any bolsters in our unit and make patient lie down flat with pressure points protected.

The scanning of kidney begins with the posterior axillary line and the first structure to be visualised is the posterior calyx which is the target. After the skin incision, the puncture needle is advanced towards the calyx using the reference of electronic puncture guide (Fig. 2.3). Care is taken to visualise the needle and the kidney all the time during the scanning. The final position of the needle is confirmed by return of urine from the needle after removing the stilette [9].

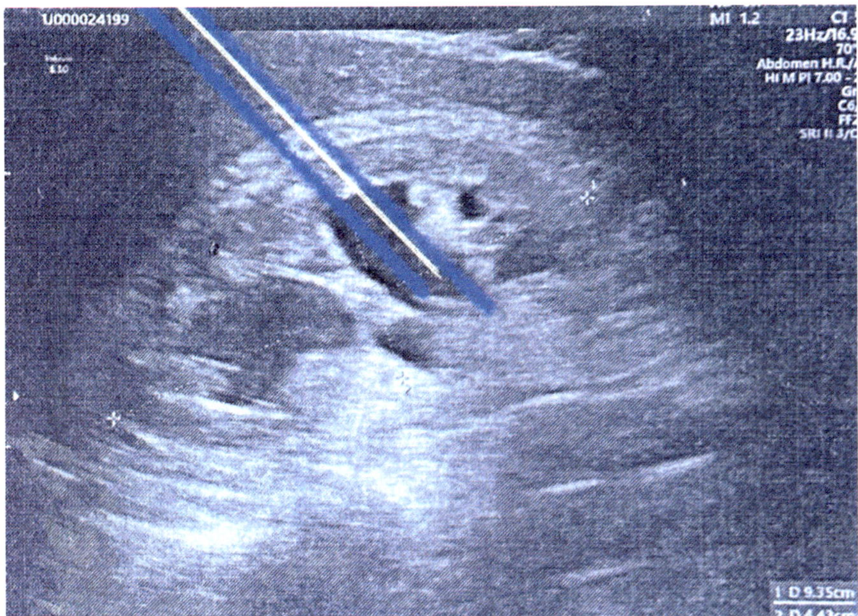

Fig. 2.3 Renal ultrasound used for percutaneous puncture. The two blue lines are the electronic guide for puncture needle (which is seen as the white line)

2.14 Trouble Shooting

If the needle tip is not seen on screening, assume a non-alignment of needle and the ultrasound probe. A biopsy guide with attachment helps a long way. Sometimes the needle does not show itself so well then it is advisable to shake the needle so as to see it as an echo reflective object.

A scored needle as already mentioned or a large bore needle helps solve these problems.

In the event that a sophisticated equipment is not available, a thin Chiba or long spinal needle is inserted para spinally in the kidney with ultrasonic guidance and then the system is opacified using contrast agent. A suitable calyx puncture can then be made completing the above steps for access. This method however is best suited for hydronephrotic or large sized kidneys.

Indications of use of ultrasound for renal access

1. In all cases needing access when suitable equipment is available
2. Special situations such as ectopic kidneys
3. Horse shoe kidney
4. Pregnancy
5. Case where retrograde access is not possible
6. When used with Doppler to visualise the vessels in abnormal position
7. Obstructed renal units post-transplant and in cases of pelvic malignancies

What's better? The ultrasound guided access or the image intensifier based access?

The use of ultrasound minimises the use of radiation and works as a useful adjunct to the modalities using X-rays. It allows visualisation of the surrounding structure and can safely be used in paediatric population as well as pregnant patients.

The use of ultrasound needs special training and sophisticated equipment and has a steep learning curve.

An image intensifier uses X-rays and gains access to renal collecting system. It however cannot locate and visualise other viscera and organs surrounding the kidneys. All studies using this technique and comparing that with use of ultrasound have shown similar safety and stone retrieval percentages [10].

2.15 Concluding Remarks

Ultrasound and image intensifier techniques both play a vital role in percutaneous renal surgery and are complimentary to each other. A modern urologist should be well versed with both so as to be able to help all possible clinical situations in s\ routine as well as complex stone surgeries.

2.16 Newer Modalities

A 3D CT scan or spiral or Axial or Coronal Maximum Intensity Projection (MIP) scans have unmatched accuracy for anatomic description. They are in use for access related to percutaneous renal surgery with almost 100% accuracy. They are known to be associated with acceptable minor (1–14%) as well as less major complications such as bleeding when compared to other modalities of access [11]. CT guided access was first reported by Haaga in 1977 [12]. It has been widely used and popularised by radiologists with the advent of refinements in CT scan equipment.

2.16.1 Indications

1. Abnormal renal anatomy such as horse shoe or renal ectopia
2. Abnormal vasculature
3. Complex stones, large bulky stone burden
4. Anatomic abnormalities such as retro renal colon [13]
5. Obesity
6. Transplant kidney
7. Failed access using other modalities

2.16.2 The Technique

It is performed in suite having dual facilities for CT as well as C arm. In the absence of such unit, multiple sequences are done with interrupted scans to limit radiation exposure to the staff.

A non-contrast CT scan is done as scout tomogram to note the position, dilation of renal pelvicalyceal system, abnormal organs around the kidney such as retro renal colon. Relation of the kidney to liver and spleen and diaphragm is noted. As scans are done, an external marker is placed to mark the skin entry just opposite the posterior calyx. Such an approach minimises the risk of bleeding as compared to the entry in infundibular region or via the pelvis. After the localisation is done, an external skin entry is marked and parts are painted, prepared and draped. A local anaesthetic is infiltrated and 18 G needle Cook™ or a Kellett needle (Rocket Medical UK™ is inserted in the target calyx). The correct entry is confirmed by aspiration of urine as clear fluid. A subsequent passage of 0.035 inch secures the access and dilation is done with PTFE dilators allowing the insertion and maintenance of nephrostomy tube.

An overview of diagnostic imaging for renal stone disease.

2.17 Preoperative Imaging for PCNL

Imaging is required for assessing stone burden. It helps plan access and gives understanding of anatomy of kidney as well as surrounding organs.

2.17.1 Plain X-Ray (KUB)

KUB helps operating surgeon to know if stone is radiopaque or not. The stone having composition of calcium oxalate monohydrate and brushite are the most opaque. Calcium oxalate monohydrate and calcium apatite sones are having intermediate opacity. Cystine and struvite stones are faintly opaque. Pure uric acid stones and the indinavir stones are radiolucent. In reality, stones have a mixed composition and are rarely diagnosed on their appearance alone.

X-rays are inexpensive and easily available but lack the sensitivity (about 58–68%) for KUB region [14] and non-availability of anatomic details of kidney and surrounding organs make it less useful in practice.

2.17.2 X-Ray IVU

Traditionally contrast enhanced imaging has been used in patients with normal renal function and has the advantage of delineating the pelvicalyceal anatomy in supine position (Fig. 2.4). This allows the surgeon to plan puncture and approach such as supracostal or other access from lower posterior calyx as per location of stones. It gives a detailed account of abnormalities such as calyceal diverticula and abnormal position of the kidney such as rotation or ascent abnormalities as pelvic or ectopic kidney. It has therefore been called the gold standard of renal imaging for acute renal colic [15].

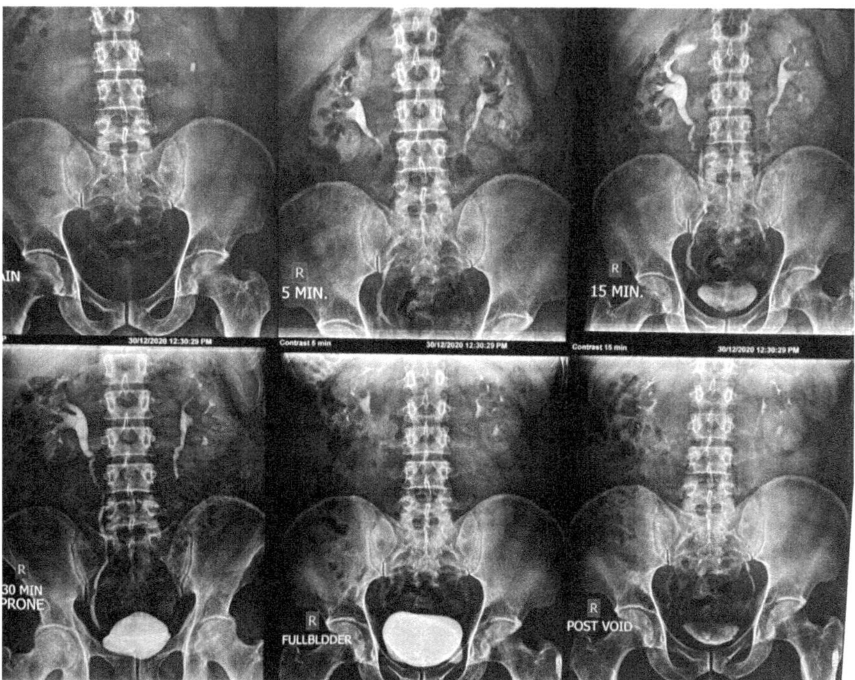

Fig. 2.4 IVU sequence in a case of lower calyx stone

2.18 CT Scan and 3D Reconstruction Imaging for Renal Stones

Non-contrast CT and CT IVU have shown very high sensitivity 94–100% and specificity of 94–97% for ureteral calculi [16]. CT allows much better delineation of anatomy of renal collecting system and hence the choice of calyx for puncture (Fig. 2.5). It gives the advantage of imaging of other organs surrounding the kidney and helps avoid accidental injury to other organs and viscera [17]. CT reconstruction allows assessment of proximity of renal calyx to pleura and lung. Hopper et al. found injury to pleura in 24% patients on the right side and 14% on the left side in end expiration. They also concluded that approach from higher up say 10th or 11th intercostal space is high with potential to injure lungs and liver and spleen especially in full inspiration [18].

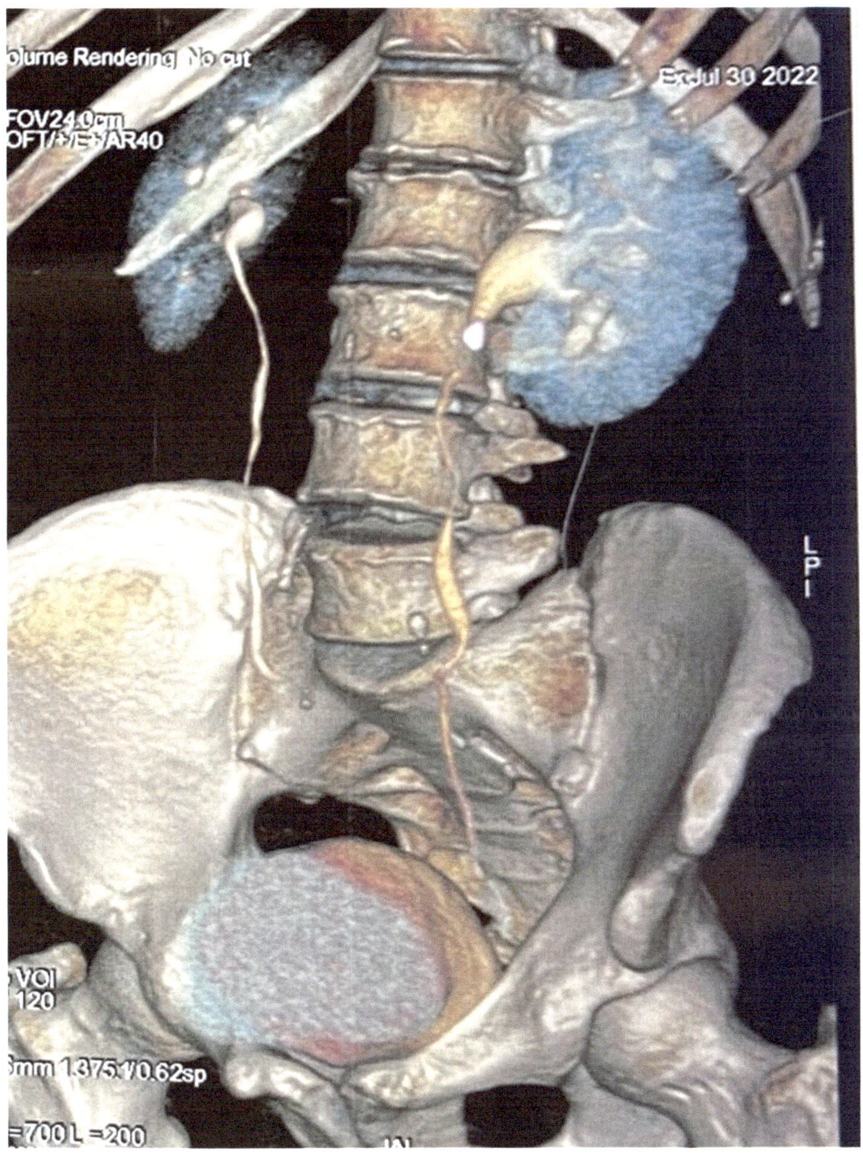

Fig. 2.5 CT IVU showing detailed anatomic reconstruction in case of left PUJ calculus. Please note the degree of dilation of PCS and anatomic details of ureter and bladder

2.19 Postoperative Imaging Following PCNL (Also Refer to Chapter on Residual Stones)

Postoperative imaging serves as an important step in assessing the success of surgery. Plain X-ray and screening just at the end of procedure using fluoroscopy reveal residual stones and allow planning of second look procedure or additional measures as ESWL subsequently.

2.19.1 Plain X-Ray KUB

Historically X-rays and nephrotomograms have been the modality of choice due to ease of availability and low cost. They have become less popular due to the drawbacks of poor sensitivity and an overestimation of stone free rates ranging from 35 to 17%, respectively. This has been compared to the gold standard, i.e. second look nephroscopy with flexible nephroscope [19].

2.19.2 Antegrade Nephrostogram

This serves as a good tool to see for clearance of stones as contrast is pushed from the PCN tube and the drainage is seen dynamically on X-ray or image intensifier. Any residual stones seen as filling defects would prompt for second line of treatment mainly relook nephroscopy or ESWL as follow-up treatment. Air bubbles and blood clots would sometimes give a false positive test and would have to be interpreted carefully. Figure 2.6a, b showing sequences of contrast injection through PCN tube and drainage film showing delineation of lower ureter.

2.19.3 Ultrasound

Ease of availability and use in various clinical situations such as abnormal anatomy, safety in pregnancy, portability make this a good accessory imaging during screening for postoperative status in PCNL patients. Operator variability and lack of reproducibility and variable image quality make this modality less reliable especially in the hands of novice operators.

2.19.4 CT KUB

Plain CT without contrast with reconstruction has been the new gold standard of imaging for residual stone estimate. It allows precise determination of size of stones and their exact location in relation to the PCN tract. Pearle et al. in their study compared CT scan X-ray KUB with the flexible nephroscopy in post PCNL patients and found CT sensitivity of 100% specificity of 64% when compared with X-rays

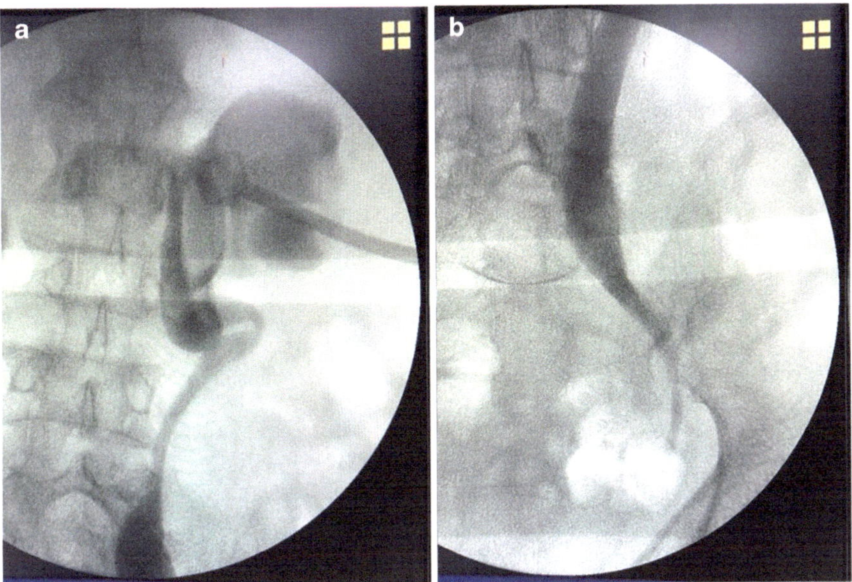

Fig. 2.6 (**a**) Contrast being injected through nephrostomy. (**b**) PCN gram showing stone free status as contrast drains down the lower ureter

showing 46% and 82% [20]. A study comprising of 147 patients by Memarsadghi et al. showed equivalent sensitivity and specificity for cuts 1.5 mm and 3 mm with dose of 11.4 mGy. They however could show that 5 mm cuts would lead to higher frequency of missed stones putting ideal cut size to 3 mm to effectively identify smaller stones. There is however no consensus on size of residual stones after PCNL [21].

There are studies suggesting difference of opinions as regards estimates of size of stones by urologists and radiologists which can be attributed to guestimates while measuring the stones as opposed to use of electronic rulers. The measured transverse diameters have been comparable on X-ray KUB and CT scan but the scans overestimated stone length by 30%. Despite these inaccuracies, CT remains the new gold standard for renal stones.

2.20 Conclusion

Radiology tools such as X-rays, ultrasonography and CT scan form the mainstay of percutaneous renal surgery.

Plain X-ray and X-ray IVU have been the major tools since many decades but ultrasound and CT scan have been more sensitive and specific tools allowing the understanding of the renal anatomy in relation to stone disease and have become very contemporary. They play a vital role in intraoperative scenario and even post-operatively to assess patient for stone free status.

References

1. Goodwin WE, Casey WC, Woolf W. Percutaneous trocar needle nephrostomy hydronephrosis. JAMA. 1955;157:891.
2. Smith AD. Smith's textbook of endourology. Raleigh: PMPH; 2007. p. 1026.
3. Fernström I, Johansson B. Percutaneous pyelolithotomy. Scand J Urol Nephrol. 1976;10(3):257–9.
4. Alken P, Hutschenreiter G, Günther R, Marberger M. Percutaneous stone manipulation. J Urol. 1981;125(4):463–6.
5. Smith AD, Reinke DB, Miller RP, Lange PH. Percutaneous nephrostomy in the management of ureteral and renal calculi. Radiology. 1979;133(1):49–54.
6. Miller NL, Matlaga BR, Lingeman JE. Techniques for fluoroscopic percutaneous renal access. J Urol. 2007;178(1):15–23.
7. Mues E, Gutiérrez J, Loske AM. Percutaneous renal access: a simplified approach. J Endourol. 2007;21(11):1271–6.
8. Singla M, Srivastava A, Kapoor R, Gupta N, Ansari MS, Dubey D, et al. Aggressive approach to staghorn calculi—safety and efficacy of multiple tracts percutaneous nephrolithotomy. Urology. 2008;71(6):1039–42.
9. Li X, Long Q, Chen X, Dalin H, He H. Real-time ultrasound-guided PCNL using a novel SonixGPS needle tracking system. Urolithiasis. 2014;42(4):341–6.
10. Ng FC, Yam WL, Lim TYB, Teo JK, Ng KK, Lim SK. Ultrasound-guided percutaneous nephrolithotomy: advantages and limitations. Investig Clin Urol. 2017;58(5):346.
11. Radecka E, Brehmer M, Holmgren K, Magnusson A. Complications associated with percutaneous nephrolithotripsy: supra- versus subcostal access: a retrospective study. Acta Radiol. 2003;44(4):447–51.
12. Haaga JR, Zelch M, Alfidi R, Stewart B, Daugherty J. CT-guided antegrade pyelography and percutaneous nephrostomy. Am J Roentgenol. 1977;128(4):621–4.
13. Skoog SJ, Reed MD, Gaudier FA, Dunn NP. The posterolateral and the retrorenal colon: implication in percutaneous stone extraction. J Urol. 1985;134(1):110–2.
14. Jackman SV, Potter SR, Regan F, Jarrett TW. Plain abdominal X-ray versus computerized tomography screening: sensitivity for stone localization after nonenhanced spiral computerized tomography. J Urol. 2000;164(2):308–10.
15. Mutazindwa T, Husseini T. Imaging in acute renal colic: the intravenous urogram remains the gold standard. Eur J Radiol. 1996;23(3):238–40.
16. Pfister SA, Deckart A, Laschke S, Dellas S, Otto U, Buitrago C, et al. Unenhanced helical computed tomography vs intravenous urography in patients with acute flank pain: accuracy and economic impact in a randomized prospective trial. Eur Radiol. 2003;13(11):2513–20.
17. Hubert J, Blum A, Cormier L, Claudon M, Regent D, Mangin P. Three-dimensional CT-scan reconstruction of renal calculi. Eur Urol. 1997;31:297–301.
18. Hopper KD, Yakes W. The posterior intercostal approach for percutaneous renal procedures: risk of puncturing the lung, spleen, and liver as determined by CT. AJR Am J Roentgenol. 1990;154:115–7.
19. Denstedt JD, Clayman RV, Picus DD. Comparison of endoscopic and radiological residual fragment rate following percutaneous nephrolithotripsy. J Urol. 1991;145(4):703–5.
20. Pearle MS, Watamull LM, Mullican MA. Sensitivity of noncontrast helical computerized tomography and plain film radiography compared to flexible nephroscopy for detecting residual fragments after percutaneous nephrostolithotomy. J Urol. 1999;162(1):23–6.
21. Memarsadeghi M, Heinz-Peer G, Helbich TH, Schaefer-Prokop C, Kramer G, Scharitzer M, et al. Unenhanced multi-detector row CT in patients suspected of having urinary stone disease: effect of section width on diagnosis. Radiology. 2005;235(2):530–6.

3 Preoperative Workup for Percutaneous Renal Surgery

Chetan Kulkarni and Subodh R. Shivde

3.1 History

PCNL is percutaneous nephrolithotomy or percutaneous nephrolithotripsy. The technique of PCNL is established well over 50 years now. Over the years, it has undergone numerous advances in its techniques and instruments and has become a safe surgical intervention modality today. Rupel and Brown [1] were the first to establish a nephrostomy tract. Fernstrom and Johansson [2] performed the first PCNL under radiological guidance.

Alken et al. [3] and Wickham [4] were the earliest proponents of the safety and efficacy of PCNL in clearing small as well as large renal pelvic calculi.

3.2 Introduction

There are many published guidelines for the treatment of renal stones but the most referred ones are the EAU and AUA guidelines [5, 6]. They have a wider set of inclusion and exclusion criteria and are comprehensive. They have also published the various levels of evidence (LE) and level of grade (LG) in these helping the practitioners understand the applications.

We would have to take into consideration the patient factors and patients' aspirations out of the surgical procedures as the outcomes would matter to both the operating surgeon and patients.

C. Kulkarni
Kolhapur, Maharashtra, India

S. R. Shivde (✉)
Department of Urology, Deenanath Mangeshkar Hospital and Research Centre, Pune, Maharashtra, India

S. R. Shivde (ed.), *Techniques in Percutaneous Renal Stone Surgery*, https://doi.org/10.1007/978-981-19-9418-0_3

Before we start the evaluation of a stone patient, we need to take into consideration some factors such as stone volume, stone composition, stone location and multicentricity of stone disease. This would help plan the desired approach well in advance and keep the operation room facilities ready with necessary equipment.

Let us see the common indications for the treatment of renal stones.

3.3 Indications for PCNL Ref. [5]

- **AUA (American Urological Association) Guidelines**
- **Renal calculi >2 cm**
- **Lower calyx stones >1 cm**
- **Calculi in diverticulum**
- **Staghorn calculi**

Indications for active stone removal (PCNL) (EAU 2016) Ref. [6, 7]

1. **Stone growth**
2. **Stone size >1.5 cm**
3. **High risk stone formers**
4. **Obstruction/symptomatic/comorbidities**
5. **Infection**
6. **Renal insufficiency**
7. **Professions (e.g. pilot)/travel**
8. **Low likelihood of spontaneous passage or failed observation/conservative treatment**

3.4 Contraindications for the PCNL Surgery

- **EAU 2018**
- **Patient on anticoagulation.**
- **Untreated UTI.**
- **Tumour in the access tract area.**
- **Potentially malignant kidney tumour.**
- **Pregnancy.**

3.5 History Taking

A detailed history should be obtained as regards bleeding diathesis, history of renal calculus disease or intervention for the same. History of allergy or hypersensitivity to contrast media or drugs in general should be obtained. The emphasis should be on choosing the best suited preoperative radiology evaluation avoiding complications such as drug hypersensitivity due to ionic or non-ionic contrast media. Due consideration should be given to the use of newer imaging forms such as non-contrast CT scan and ultrasonography combined with it to evaluate patients with high risk or those in need of repeated surgeries. Previous history of urinary tract infections and treatment taken should be listed. In case of a female patient, a history of last menstrual period and a possible urinary pregnancy test would help rule out pregnancy in a concurrent stone scenario.

3.5.1 Physical Examination

A relevant physical examination of abdomen and back with genitalia is a must to rule out access related problems such as scarred back, paraspinal area and congenital problems such as kyphosis or scoliosis. This would have to be taken into consideration for the choice of operative procedure and the approach whether supine or prone.

3.5.2 Laboratory Tests as Pre-operative Workup

Bleeding/clotting parameters
Prothrombin time (PT) and International Normalised Ratio (INR)
Activated partial thromboplastin time (APTT)
Platelet count

Renal function tests
Blood urea nitrogen
Serum Creatinine
Serum electrolytes
E-(Glomerular Filtration Rate) GFR.

3.5.3 Complete Blood Cell Count

Any parameter suggestive of anaemia would have to be worked up prior and necessary arrangement be made for blood or blood products. Platelet abnormalities to be noted and corrected duely, given the higher risk of bleeding involved in the surgery.

3.5.4 Urine Analysis and Urine Culture

It is imperative that the urine is sterile prior to an elective PCNL scenario and a pretreatment urine analysis including culture sensitivity is a must. Any pre-existing infection should be treated with a suitable antibiotic course. The procedure is covered with appropriate doses as per institutional protocol.

3.5.5 Imaging

Historically plain X-ray KUB and X-ray IVU were the mainstay of pre-operative workup. While the following list needs a consideration depending on the presentation of the patient and clinical scenario, a CT KUB is considered the new norm for pre-op evaluation of a stone patient [5].

- **Ultrasound with X-ray KUB (NO FUNCTIONAL INFORMATION OBTAINED)**
- **Intravenous pyelography (GOOD ANATOMICAL AND FUNCTIONAL STUDY)**
- **Retrograde pyelography (ON TABLE ANATOMY ROAD MAP)**
- **CT scan with intravenous contrast (CURRENT GOLD STANDARD FOR STRUCTURAL AND FUNCTIONAL WORK UP)**
- **MRI**
- **Nuclear renography**

Role of nuclear medicine imaging needs appropriate clinical judgement in cases where medical conditions or comorbidity factors are likely to further deteriorate glomerular filtration rate (GFR) leading to the worsening of renal parameters. It would also help in bilateral stone disease to choose the side to operate upon first. The worse side with deteriorating function would then be a priority.

Additional data collection to be done with the use of the following charts or nomograms. These help us understand the complexity of the stone disease and measure the outcomes following surgical procedures as regards success, i.e. stone free rates, and evaluation of complications following surgery. They would form an integral part of modern-day urology practice in future [8–10].

3.6 Guy's Stone Scoring (GSS) System Ref. [8]

This system scores the complexity of PCNL. It is used to predict the success of the procedure. It has been widely used to predict stone free rates of the procedure.

- **Grade 1**—Thus incudes stone in kidney pelvis and or mid and lower calyx stone solitary stone in mid/lower calyx
- **Grade 2**—Stones in kidney with normal anatomy, stones in upper calyx

- Single stone in kidney with abnormal anatomy
- **Grade 3**—Multiple stones in kidney with normal anatomy, Calyceal diverticulum stones
- **Grade 4**—Complete staghorn calculus

Hasan et al. in their study using the GSS based on IVU showed that it is a good easy-to-use tool. It helped them predict early success rates and also the complications when performing PCNL through upper calyx [11].

3.6.1 S.T.O.N.E. Morphometry

S.T.O.N.E. score predicts the success of treatment and the risk of perioperative complications of PCNL [9].

Size of calculus:	0–4 mm	(1)
	4–8 mm	(2)
	8–16 mm	(3)
	>16 mm	(4)
Tract length:	<10 cm	(1)
	>10 cm	(2)
Obstruction—hydroureteronephrosis (HUN)		
	Mild HUN	(1)
	Moderate/severe	(2)
Number of calyces:	1–2	(1)
	3	(2)
Staghorn		(3)
Essence:	<950	(1)
(STONE DENSITY)	>950	(3)

3.6.2 CROES Nomogram

CROES (Clinical Research Office of the Endourological Society) nomogram accurately predicts stone complexity and postoperative efficacy [10].

It takes into consideration

1. Stone burden:
   (a) Length in mm
   (b) Width in mm
   (c) Stone burden = 0.785 length/width
   (d) Add individual burdens if multiple stones
2. Calyceal location: position in renal pelvis and number of calyces

3. Stone count: single or multiple

Aminsharifi et al. compared a new software using machine learning with the established methods of stone assessment such as the GSS and CROES nomogram [12].

In their institutional audit of 146 patients undergoing PCNL, they studied the actual outcomes using all three methods. A receiver operating curve (ROC) was generated for all three methods, and the area under curve (AUC) was calculated. The AUC for software was (0.95) significantly greater than AUC for GSS (0.615) and for CROES nomogram (0.62), (p value less than 0.001). This suggests an accuracy of 80–95% for newer tools such as machine learning. The authors strongly suggest validating these tools against the external sources of prediction.

Lai et al. compared four methods of stone morphometry and found that all predicted stone free status accurately. In their study of 349 patients comparing multiple methods, they found the SeREC (Seoul National University Renal Stone Complexity) scoring system to be more predictable and easier to implement. They however concluded that none of the methods accurately predicted the complications in the studied cohort [13].

Kailavasan et al. in their systematic review of paediatric stone patients undergoing PCNL found the CROES nomograms to be more accurate and supportive of the outcomes and GUY'S nomogram showing least accuracy. The interstudy variability and differences in recording of variables such as the different criteria for stone free rates were responsible for the differences [14].

References

1. Rupel E, Brown R. Nephroscopy with removal of stone following nephrostomy for obstructive calculous anuria. J Urol. 1941;46:177–82. https://doi.org/10.1016/S0022-5347(17)70906-8.
2. Fernström I, Johansson B. Percutaneous pyelolithotomy. Scand J Urol Nephrol. 1976;10:257–9. https://doi.org/10.1080/21681805.1976.11882084.
3. Alken P, Hutschenreiter G, Günther R, Marberger M. Percutaneous stone manipulation. J Urol. 2017;197:S154–7. https://doi.org/10.1016/j.juro.2016.10.070.
4. Jones DJ, Russell GL, Kellett MJ, Wickham JEA. The changing practice of percutaneous stone surgery. Review of 1000 cases 1981–1988. Br J Urol. 1990;66:1–5. https://doi.org/10.1111/j.1464-410X.1990.tb14852.x.
5. Assimos D, Krambeck A, Miller NL, Manoj Monga M, Murad H, Nelson CP, Pace KT, Pais VM, Pearle MS, Preminger GM, Razvi H, Shah O, Matlaga BR. Surgical management of stones: American Urological Association/Endourological Society Guideline, PART I. J Urol. 2016;196:1153–60. https://doi.org/10.1016/j.juro.2016.05.090.
6. Bultitude M, Smith D, THOMAS K. Contemporary management of stone disease: the new EAU urolithiasis guidelines for 2015. Eur Urol. 2016;69:483–4. https://doi.org/10.1016/j.eururo.2015.08.010.
7. Türk C, Petřík A, Sarica K, Seitz C, Skolarikos A, Straub M, Knoll T. EAU guidelines on interventional treatment for urolithiasis. Eur Urol. 2016;69:475–82. https://doi.org/10.1016/j.eururo.2015.07.041.
8. Thomas K, Smith NC, Hegarty N, et al. The Guy's stone score—grading the complexity of percutaneous nephrolithotomy procedures. Urology. 2011;78:277–81.

9. Okhunov Z, Friedlander JI, George AK, Duty BD, Moreira DM, Srinivasan AK, Hillelsohn J, Smith AD, Okeke Z. S.T.O.N.E. nephrolithometry: novel surgical classification system for kidney calculi. Urology. 2013;81(6):1154–60.
10. Sfoungaristos S, Gofrit ON, Yutkin VL, Landau EH, Pode D, Duvdevani M. External validation of CROES nephrolithometry as a preoperative predictive system for percutaneous nephrolithotomy outcomes. J Urol. 2016;195(2):372–6. https://doi.org/10.1016/j.juro.2015.08.079.
11. Hasan A, Singh G, Panda S. Intravenous pyelogram (IVP)-based Guy's Stone Score (GSS) utility for prediction of outcomes of upper pole access percutaneous nephrolithotomy (PCNL). Nephro-Urol Mon. 2022;14(2):e121179. https://brieflands.com/articles/num-121179.html#abstract
12. Aminsharifi A, Irani D, Tayebi S, Jafari Kafash T, Shabanian T, Parsaei H. Predicting the postoperative outcome of percutaneous nephrolithotomy with machine learning system: software validation and comparative analysis with Guy's stone score and the CROES nomogram. J Endourol. 2020;34(6):692–9.
13. Lai S, Jiao B, Jiang Z, Liu J, Seery S, Chen X, et al. Comparing different kidney stone scoring systems for predicting percutaneous nephrolithotomy outcomes: a multicenter retrospective cohort study. Int J Surg. 2020;81:55–60.
14. Kailavasan M, Berridge C, Yuan Y, Turner A, Donaldson J, Biyani CS. A systematic review of nomograms used in urolithiasis practice to predict clinical outcomes in paediatric patients. J Pediatr Urol. 2022;18(4):448–62. https://www.sciencedirect.com/science/article/pii/S147751312200211X

Consent for PCNL

4

Consent for Percutaneous Renal Stone Procedure: A Dialogue Between Patient and Treating Urosurgeon

Lalit Shah and Subodh R. Shivde

As the adage goes *"The consent for a procedure is not worth the piece of paper it's written on"*

A surgeon should dutifully explain in a simple round of talks or consultation, the current medical status, the need for surgery, the best form of operative procedure and other alternative therapies if any. Also having explained the surgical therapies, the doctor would have to get the patient to understand the possibility of major or minor complications or adverse outcomes.

In an informed consent (IC) or the standard verbal consent (SVC), the patient and relatives of patient can go home with some written information or some references to the operative procedure via internet resources and should be able to return with the signed consent. Queries if any should be handled by the operative team and leave room for further discussion as well. It is imperative on part of the surgeon to document this process and be able to archive it as and when necessary.

A clear and comprehensive discussion between the patient and the surgeon would lead to an authorization of percutaneous nephrolithotomy (PCNL) procedure by the patient. It would not be wise to hold a procedure or not be able to offer it due to lack of surgical expertise on part of surgeon or non-availability of suitable equipment. An operating surgeon is morally obligated to refer a patient to another more experienced or specialist endourology colleague for second opinion or even a referral to a higher volume centre if a case is complex and more demanding [1].

An ideal PCNL consent therefore would have many features to it including other alternatives to the offered surgery, the true Stone Free Rates (SFR), mention major as well as minor complications with their approximate percentages and treatment sequelae.

L. Shah (✉)
Raipur, India

S. R. Shivde
Department of Urology, Deenanath Mangeshkar Hospital and Research Centre, Pune, Maharashtra, India

S. R. Shivde (ed.), *Techniques in Percutaneous Renal Stone Surgery*, https://doi.org/10.1007/978-981-19-9418-0_4

In the current era, the medical practice especially the surgical aspect should be handled with **a patient centric or patient focused way**. The age-old ways of handling medico legal matters such as the Bolam test or Bolam principle in the United Kingdom are being further reviewed, and the focus is shifting from **medical paternalism** (the learned community opining on the way of handling the case scenario as standard or being practiced by someone) to **patient focused ways** wherein medical opinions are deemed secondary to discussion-based patient information approaches [2–4]. As more and more specialty specific bodies start demanding detailed patient information and consent as preoperative requirement, the choice of details such as percentages of complications and their commonness and sometimes explanation of their severity would make a surgeon's task more and more difficult.

As we advance in technology and medical practice, we are obliged to use better forms of communication and informed consent cannot be an exception to this. Newer apps are being developed and used by urologist which are known to improve understanding of the patients [5]. These apps, called as the portable video media (PVM)- available as iURO has been shown to be statistically better than standard verbal consent (SVC) in patients undergoing transurethral surgery. They are shown to improve patients' understanding of the disease conditions and operative procedure required. Widespread use of such apps in the stone treatment scenario is a good development to happen in the interest of both patients and doctors. This would ensure better content delivery to the patient about disease condition and available treatments, along with alternatives if any. These methods would also take the pressure off the medical system, which is under increasing stress of work burden and delivery of healthcare in the best possible way [6]. Education and health literacy are the possible factors affecting the widespread use of these methods, but these would certainly help patients and doctors get over the hurdle of deficits of the SVC such as inability to recall and make content delivery better.

Video consent as a process has been in practice for a while now, for use in complex surgeries such as laparoscopy in urology [7]. This study by the UK unit followed a protocol of verbal consenting and preoperative anaesthetic assessment followed by admission for surgery wherein the patients were shown an operative video and then video consent was done. This was shown to be an effective way of patient education and resulted in better patient satisfaction on post procedure enquiry. While the internet appears to be a big source of unsolicited medical information, the surgical community needs to channelize this good patient information with the use of services such as video consent. This would serve the dual purpose of good documentation along with better patient understanding and improved patient satisfaction. There is a definite scope for larger randomized controlled studies in this area of video consenting.

4.1 Financial Consent

It is generally believed that clinical decisions are not to be made on medical considerations alone but also on economic facts [8]. In the current scenario of escalating costs of medical treatment and surgical options, patients and doctors are under increasing pressure to cope up with the finances. A good doctor who practices ethically would have to assess his patient's financial status and the available insurance plans which decide some or most of the treatments. In the situation where patients are not able to take care of the costs, it is the moral and ethical obligation of the treating doctor and institute to guide them and refer them to public hospitals or charitable organizations, so the treatments commence without further morbidity. A doctor should include budget in the clinical decision-making process to ensure that the best possible care is offered within the available means with measurable benefit to the patient [9].

A prototype consent form for PCNL (Reproduced with permission): (Courtesy Dr. L Shah)

Date: _______________

CONSENT FOR PERCUTANEOUS NEPHROLITHOTOMY

Patient's Name : ________________s/o________________ Age/Sex--------------------------------
Address ------------------------------ h/o major illness & co-morbidities--------------------------------

1. I request to have Percutaneous nephrolithotomy (PCNL) operation to be performed under overall supervision of Dr.______________________. (Name of Urologist) & his team.
2. I have been explained about the kind of procedure he /she will perform and has answered my questions about my condition, disease process, nature and purpose of the procedure, expenditure, likelihood of success, benefits, its effect on my body, risks involved in it, possible complication, sequelae etc. in detail to my satisfaction in my language.

3. I have been explained about the risks involved and/ or likely complications in Percutaneous Nephrolithotomy (PCNL), i.e.

(A) Complications:
Bleeding (intraoperative /postoperative) requiring blood transfusion (1-10%),
Bleeding from arterio -venous fistula or pseudo-aneurysm needing angioembolisation (0.5%),
Infection and sepsis (upto2.5%),
Failed access in (less than 5%),
Perforation of renal pelvis and/or ureter (less than 2%),
Pneumothorax or pleural effusion requiring drainage (4-12%) when supracostal approach used and failure of equipment.
Possible migration of stone fragment and possibility of residual fragments/stones.
(B) I have been explained that, there is possibility of other rare complications.
(C) Very rarely there may be need for open surgical procedure, even need for nephrectomy (removal of kidney) as a last resort as a life-saving measure.
(D) Risk of injury to structures close to kidney such as Lung, Pleura, solid organs such as Liver, Spleen and Bowel structures such as colon and small bowel. In case of identification of such untoward event I give consent to my operating team to do the needful as remedial measure.

4. I have also been explained about the alternative methods of treatment i.e., medical management, Shockwave lithotripsy, other methods of surgical treatment like open pyelolithotomy, Endoscopic Renal surgery such as RIRS etc.

I have also been explained about likely consequences, if I do not agree to undergo above mentioned operation, like kidney damage, transient or permanent kidney failure, infection, septicemia, pain, development of malignancy (Cancer), harm to the other kidney and loss of life etc.

5. I understand that during the procedure, doctor may find other associated pathology in me that need correction at the same time, like narrowing of infundibula, pelviureteric obstruction etc. I authorize the doctor to perform such other procedure needed for my own benefit.

6. I have been explained about the complications related to surgery and/or anaesthesia, which may be life threatening in very few cases.

7. I have been explained that the procedure will be performed under spinal/epidural/general anaesthesia. However, sometimes change in plan may be needed, and I authorize the surgeon and anesthetist to do so in my benefit.

8. I have been explained that sonography/other imaging and laboratory tests may not always correlate with clinical judgement.

9. I have been explained and understand that blood transfusion may be needed occasionally. I give consent for the same. I understand that there may be a need for blood transfusion related complications.

10. No guarantee can be given about the outcome of the procedure as every patient has a different physiology and body response. But I have been assured of best humanly possible medicare.

11. I agree to co-operate with my doctor and his team, and to follow his/her instructions and recommendations about my care and treatment, including the management of tubes i.e.PCN and Double J stent etc. I have been advised for regular follow-up examination, avoid heavy exercises.

12. I have also been explained that any other procedure will only be carried out if it is necessary to save my life or to prevent serious harm to my health.

13. I have understood the aforesaid and I am giving my consent willingly with sound mental state without any coercion.

14. I have also been explained that in certain situations the procedure must be done as staged procedure for my own benefit.

15. I have been explained about the disease, operative procedure Percutaneous nephrolithotomy (PCNL) and anaesthesia in detail in my language to my satisfaction. (To be written by the patient in his handwriting) ____________________

Patient

Sign : .... Date: ....

Name : .... Age: ....

Address : .... Mobile No: ....

Witness

Sign : .... Date: ....

Name : .... Address:..........................

.... Mobile No: ....

CONFIRMATION OF CONSENT

I have confirmed with the patient that he/she has no further questions and wishes the procedure to go ahead.

Urologist

Sign : .... Date: ....

Name : .... Address:..........................

....

Signature of a witness

....

References

1. Segura JW, Preminger GM, Assimos DG, Dretler SP, Kahn RI, Lingeman JE, Macaluso JN, McCullough DL. Nephrolithiasis clinical guidelines panel summary report on the management of Staghorn calculi. J Urol. 1994;151:1648–51. https://doi.org/10.1016/S0022-5347(17)35330-2.
2. McCormack DJ, Gulati A, Mangwani J. Informed consent. Bone Jt J. 2018;100-B:687–92. https://doi.org/10.1302/0301-620x.100b6.bjj-2017-1542.r1.
3. The Bolam Test. https://medical-dictionary.thefreedictionary.com/Bolam+test.
4. The Bolitho test. https://medical-dictionary.thefreedictionary.com/Bolitho+test.

5. Armijos León S, Rodriguez-Rubio F, Rioja Zuazu J, Sanchez Barrios V, Caballero JG, Sanjeev B, Canelon E. MP92-04 improvement of informed consent in urological surgeries: portable video media versus standard verbal communication. A randomized controlled trial. J Urol. 2017;197:e1227. https://doi.org/10.1016/j.juro.2017.02.2865.
6. Winter M, Kam J, Nalavenkata S, Hardy E, Handmer M, Ainsworth H, Lee WG, Louie-Johnsun M. The use of portable video media vs standard verbal communication in the urological consent process: a multicentre, randomised controlled, crossover trial. BJU Int. 2016;118:823–8. https://doi.org/10.1111/bju.13595.
7. Sahai A, Kucheria R, Challacombe B, Dasgupta P. Video consent: a pilot study of informed consent in laparoscopic urology and its impact on patient satisfaction. JSLS. 2006;10(1):21–5.
8. Maynard A. Ethical issues in the economics of rationing healthcare. Br J Urol. 1995;76(Suppl 2):59–64. https://doi.org/10.1111/j.1464-410x.1995.tb07873.x.
9. Ethics in Neurosurgical Practice—Google Books. https://books.google.co.in/books?hl=en&lr=&id=iJ7bDwAAQBAJ&oi=fnd&pg=PA73&dq=Financial+consentsin+Urosurgery&ots=Qzm0j3St0O&sig=bcQUOsCavPLa_b8iU.

5 Anesthetic Considerations for Percutaneous Renal Surgery

Amruta Bedekar and Bhagyashree Shivde

Percutaneous renal stone surgery has been done under all forms of anesthesia, namely local infiltration, regional (spinal or epidural), and general anesthesia. The percutaneous renal surgeries are peculiar in a way that the patient needs varying operative positions such as lithotomy, prone position, or supine position for Endoscopic Combined Intrarenal Surgery (ECIRS). The thing which remains common for all of the above procedures is the patient and his or her comorbidities. The risk factors for complications such as sepsis, bleeding, hypothermia, and fluid overload with electrolyte imbalances remain the same. It is therefore important to understand the principles of anesthesia for this form of surgery.

5.1 Introduction

We aim to achieve the following objectives by the end of this review

1. Perioperative assessment and optimization of patient for surgery.
2. Discuss the choice of anesthetic techniques available with pros and cons of each with the patient.
3. Understand the intraoperative considerations involving the positioning of the patient, fluid management, and temperature measurements regularly to prevent complications.
4. Being aware of the possible perioperative events and complications with emphasis on the early detection and treatment.

A. Bedekar (✉) · B. Shivde
Deenanath Mangeshkar Hospital and Research Centre, Pune, India

S. R. Shivde (ed.), *Techniques in Percutaneous Renal Stone Surgery*,
https://doi.org/10.1007/978-981-19-9418-0_5

5.2 Pathophysiological Considerations

Preoperative evaluation consists of careful assessment and understanding of the complex diseases and concurrent comorbidities. The age ranges span from pediatric to geriatric groups. Patients present with large stone burden and bilateral disease with renal derangement making the conduct of anesthesia challenging. The common comorbidities include obesity, cardiovascular insufficiency, and respiratory problems.

We detail some of the problems, their implications and pertinent management in Table 5.1.

Unless a thorough perioperative evaluation and optimization of the patient is done, the surgical outcomes will not be as planned and recovery would be prolonged with increase in the morbidity and increased hospital stay. This will have an economic impact as well pushing the cost of surgery up. Table 5.2 gives perioperative planning and management of common prescription drugs.

Table 5.1 Common medical problems and their implications

Medical problem	Perioperative implication	Optimization/management
Hypertension	• Rightward shift of autoregulatory curve: hypotension may precipitate organ ischemia • Uncontrolled hypertension may increase intraoperative blood loss	• Optimization of pre-op blood pressure control • Cardiac evaluation with ECG. 2D echo, stress test, angiography if indicated • Physician input
Diabetes	• Increased risk of post-op infection, poor wound healing, hypoglycemic events	• Optimization of pre-op sugar control • Glucose/insulin management during peri-op period • Use of regional anesthesia
Cardiac disease	• Risk of perioperative cardiac event	• Cardiac risk evaluation and explanation to the patient • Physician and cardiologist input • Antiplatelet and anti-coagulant drug interactions
Thyroid disease: hyperthyroidism, hypothyroidism	• Risk of thyroid storm • Delayed recovery from anesthesia, myxedema coma	• Euthyroid status pre-op
Bronchial asthma	• Risk of intraoperative bronchospasm	• Inhalers and nebulization preoperatively • Avoidance of drugs precipitating bronchospasm • Use of regional anesthesia
Chronic kidney disease	• Delayed metabolism of drugs • Peri-op hypotension or nephrotoxic drugs may worsen renal function	• Avoid hypotension • Avoid nephrotoxic drugs • Dosage adjustment for drugs metabolized by kidney

Table 5.2 Perioperative management of common prescription drugs

Medication	Drug	Recommendation
Anti-hypertensives	Beta blocker Calcium channel blocker ACE inhibitor Angiotensin receptor blocker Diuretics	Continue Continue Withhold for 24–48 h Withhold for 24–48 h Assess fluid-electrolyte status
Anti-diabetics	Oral antihyperglycemic Insulin	Withhold during fasting period As per BSL monitoring
Cardiac medications	Nitrates Antiarrhythmics Alpha blockers Vasodilators	Continue. May need conversion to IV preparations perioperatively
Bronchodilators	Inhaled/oral	Continue. May need pre-op nebulization

5.3 Management of Patients on Antiplatelet Drugs or Anticoagulants

Percutaneous renal surgeries are likely to encounter heavy bleeding and hence continuation of this group of drugs would further increase this bleeding risk during or after surgery. Discontinuation of the drugs would cause complications such as thrombosis of coronary stents, pulmonary embolisms, and risks of ischemic events of cardiovascular and neurological systems.

Stopping of regular medications or continuation should be a joint decision between physician, cardiologist, anesthesia, and surgical teams. Figures 5.1 and 5.2 show a simple practical algorithm to stop and manage patients on aspirin and ADP inhibitors.

In case of patients on warfarin, it needs to be stopped for at least 5 days prior to surgery. The target INR should be maintained with the use of bridging therapy (heparin/unfractionated or low molecular weight heparin). This should be stopped 8 h prior to surgery. Restart warfarin as soon as possible after the surgery.

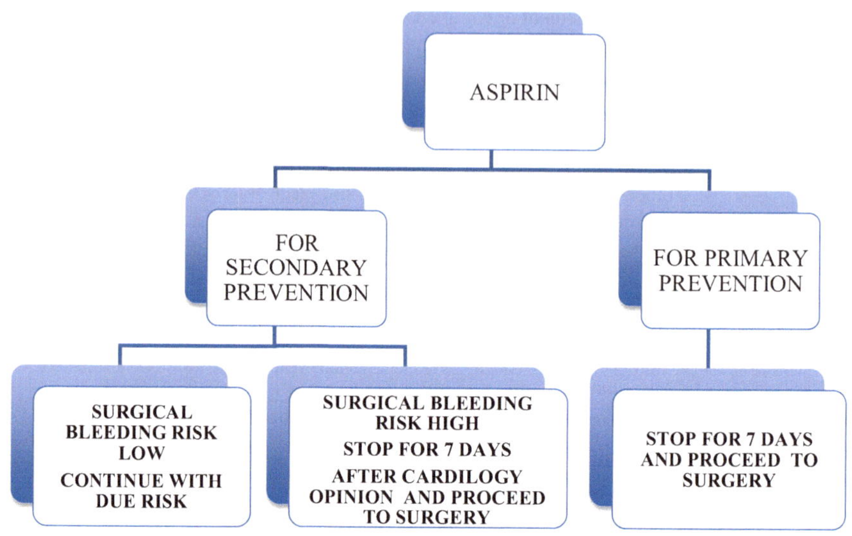

Fig. 5.1 For management of patients on aspirin (acetyl salicylic acid/ASA)

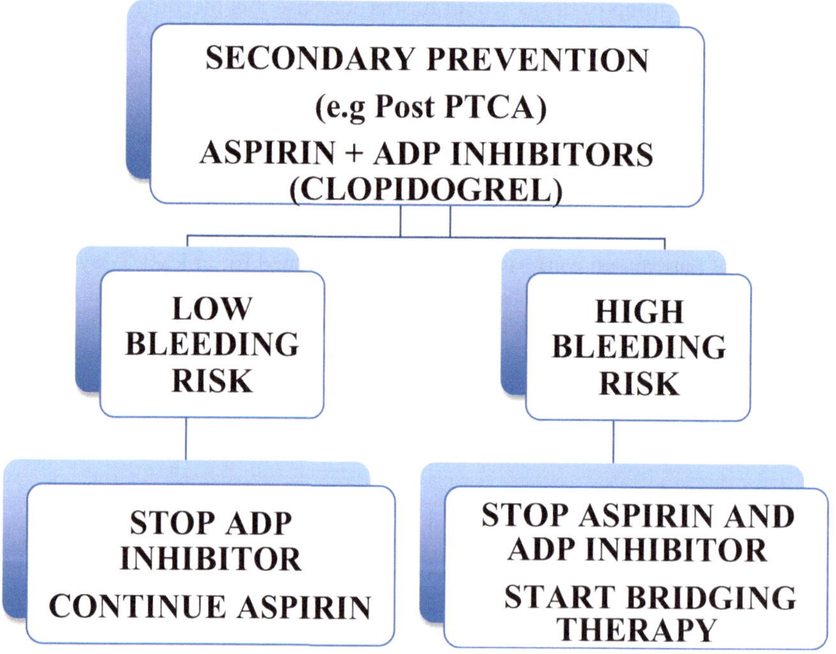

Fig. 5.2 For the management of patients on ASA + ADP INHIBITOR (adenosine diphosphate receptor antagonist)

5.4 Management of Infective Complications During and After Percutaneous Renal Surgery and the Role of Anesthesia

Urinary tract infections (UTI) are the commonest complications following percutaneous renal surgery. The factors responsible for this are associated diabetes, abnormal anatomy, increased duration of surgery, and inadequate preparation of the patient as regards antibiotic prophylaxis. Septic shock and death have been reported in approximately 1% of patients undergoing percutaneous renal surgery (Table 5.3).

We recommend the use of broad-spectrum quinolones or third-generation cephalosporins to be used prior to induction but the choice is governed by the clinical scenario and is best finalized after discussion with the surgical team.

Table 5.3 Factors increasing risk of postoperative UTI/sepsis in PCNL

Patient factors	Stone characteristics	Procedural factors
Extremes of age	Large, complex stones	Increased operative time
Diabetes	Recurrent stones	Increased number of access tracts
Obesity	Struvite stones	Larger volume of irrigation fluid
Female sex	Hydronephrosis	
	Positive pelvic urine culture	
	Positive stone culture	

Refs. [1, 2]

5.5 Technique of Anesthesia

Although a number of previous studies have compared the safety and efficacy of regional versus general anesthesia for percutaneous renal surgery, the choice of anesthesia is the result of discussion between the surgeon, the anesthetic team, and the patient [3–6].

Percutaneous renal surgeries could be performed safely under regional anesthesia, i.e., spinal or epidural; due consideration should be given to the duration of procedure, comfort of the patient in prone position and also the fact that the patient will be fully awake. There would be significant difficulty in accessing the airway and securing it in a prone position. This adds to the difficulties of sedation of the patient and also bring about the changes in position of patient, say from lithotomy to prone position if regional preferred. Regional anesthesia has been used for percutaneous renal stone surgery but patient may feel uncomfortable due to long duration of procedure and may need epidural infusion. It may be significantly difficult to assess the level of block during the surgery [7, 8].

We recommend general anesthesia, tracheal intubation with controlled ventilation. This allows the patient to be kept immobile during the entire duration of the procedure. This also allows our surgical team to have a controlled ventilation during the initial puncture and sometimes during the retrieval of stone fragments from inaccessible parts of the pelvicalyceal system. We prefer to give relaxant at the time of initial puncture and pain relief at the time of tract dilation.

5.6 Preparation of the Patient for Percutaneous Renal Surgery Ref. [9]

1. Patient positioning

Key Points

1. Care required in changing patients position from supine/lithotomy to prone position
2. Adequate man power required to shift the patient
3. Care of pressure points and adequate care of knee and hip positioning especially in patients with previous joint surgeries
4. Avoiding pressure on the vulnerable parts such as face and eyes
5. Position induced neuropraxia would have to be avoided

All of the above extra precautions would be avoided in case of supine PCNL, i.e., ECRIS.

Patient would have less changes in position and the patient's breathing would be free of difficulty.

5.7 Intraoperative Considerations

5.7.1 Theater and Anesthesia Preparation

A considerably large space is needed for such surgeries as there is an expected crowding of space with equipment such as image intensifier, video trolley, cart carrying lithotripsy device. Due considerations would have to be given during the planning of theater space. The need for longer tubings for the ventilator and extensions of the intravenous tubings and monitoring leads would have been planned. Table 5.4 gives a simple planning and treatment model for common intraoperative problems during percutaneous renal surgery.

Table 5.4 Intraoperative clinical problems and remedial measures

Clinical problem	Remedy
Hypothermia caused by ambient temperature and surface cooling	1. Rectal/esophageal probe 2. Warmed fluids and irrigation 3. Patient warming devices, e.g., blankets and sleeves
Pyrexia caused by release of endotoxins	1. Good appropriate antibiotics used preoperatively 2. Antipyretics
Blood loss (difficult to assess due to use of large volume of irrigation fluids)	1. Early rapid assessment of Hb/PCV 2. Preoperative group and saving of sample of blood and early transfusion for significant loss
Fluid and electrolyte imbalances	Preoperative central venous access and or good IV access

5.8 Postoperative Care of Percutaneous Renal Surgery Patients

1. Careful monitoring of vitals of the patient with specific emphasis on watching for tachycardia and hypotension (bleeding or impending sepsis), tachypnoea, reduced SpO_2 (possible atelectasis, fluid in the pleural space or pneumothorax). It is vital to rule out pneumothorax in cases of higher intercostal punctures. While in the operating room, use the image intensifier and in doubtful cases we strongly recommend a chest X-ray in sitting position in the recovery room.
2. While in the recovery phase, patients do complain of mild to moderate pain at the operation site and we recommend using paracetamol or codeine derivatives.
3. Monitoring of the urine output as regards volume and color to note ongoing hematuria.
4. We recommend a strict watch in case of profuse hematuria seen in per-urethral catheter or the PCN tube and call the surgical team. Due consideration is given to the replacement of blood in case abnormal laboratory values are seen during the postoperative period. An early clamping of the PCN tube is recommended by our surgical team in case of brisk hemorrhage.

References

1. Korets R, Graversen JA, Kates M, Mues AC, Gupta M. Post-percutaneous nephrolithotomy systemic inflammatory response: a prospective analysis of preoperative urine, renal pelvic urine and stone cultures. J Urol. 2011;186:1899–903. https://doi.org/10.1016/j.juro.2011.06.064.
2. Seymour CW, Liu VX, Iwashyna TJ, et al. Assessment of clinical criteria for sepsis: for the third international consensus definitions for sepsis and septic shock (sepsis-3). JAMA. 2016;315(8):762–74. https://doi.org/10.1001/jama.2016.0288.
3. Chen Y, Zhou Z, Sun W, et al. Minimally invasive percutaneous nephrolithotomy under peritubal local infiltration anaesthesia. World J Urol. 2011;29:773–7.
4. Parikh GP, Shah VR, Modi MP, et al. The analgesic efficacy of peritubal infiltration of 0.25% bupivacaine in percutaneous nephrolithotomy—a prospective randomised study. J Anesthesiol Clin Pharmacol. 2011;27:481–4.
5. Kuzgunbay B, Turunc T, Akin S, et al. Percutaneous nephrolithotomy under general versus combined spinal epidural anaesthesia. J Endourol. 2009;23:1835–8.
6. Singh V, Sinha RJ, Sankhwar SN, et al. A prospective randomised study comparing percutaneous nephrolithotomy under combined spinal epidural anaesthesia with percutaneous nephrolithotomy under general anaesthesia. Urol Int. 2011;87:293–8.
7. Rozentsveig V, Neulander EZ, Roussabrov E, et al. Anaesthetic considerations during percutaneous nephrolithotomy. J Clin Anesth. 2007;19:351–5.
8. Malik I, Wadhwa R. Percutaneous nephrolithotomy: current clinical opinions and anesthesiologists perspective. Anesthesiol Res Pract. 2016;2016:9036872. https://doi.org/10.1155/2016/9036872.
9. Checketts MR, Alladi R, Ferguson K, Gemmell L, Handy JM, Klein AA, Love NJ, Misra U, Morris C, Nathanson MH, Rodney GE, Verma R, Pandit JJ. Recommendations for standards of monitoring during anaesthesia and recovery 2015: Association of Anaesthetists of Great Britain and Ireland. Anaesthesia. 2016;71:85–93. https://doi.org/10.1111/anae.13316.

PCNL Armamentarium: Rigid and Flexible Nephroscopes

6

Rohan Valsangkar and Jaydeep Date

6.1 Nephroscopes

Nephroscope is an optical instrument for inspection of renal pelvicalyceal system by percutaneous approach and for the performance of therapeutic procedures (mainly PCNL).

6.2 History

The very first nephroscopy was performed by Rupel and Brown. They did this by ingenious way by placing a rigid cystoscope through a nephrostomy tract to remove stones. The credit of removing stones percutaneously under radiological control however goes to Fernström and Johansson. In 1976, they also published a method of dilating the tract using polythene dilators and extraction of stones percutaneously using Dormia basket. The historical cystoscopes used for renal stone extraction were replaced by rigid nephroscopes having larger channels.

Nephroscopes can be classified in a variety of ways. They could be rigid or flexible. Karl Storz introduced the rigid nephroscope in 1965. It was the first instrument used for viewing the pyelocaliceal system. The various types available are with rod lens system and with optical fibres.

R. Valsangkar (✉) · J. Date
Deenanath Mangeshkar Hospital, Pune, India

S. R. Shivde (ed.), *Techniques in Percutaneous Renal Stone Surgery*, https://doi.org/10.1007/978-981-19-9418-0_6

6.2.1 Rigid Scope Design and Principle of Optics

It uses a system of Hopkins rod lenses along a tunnel to relay an image to eyepiece. The image magnification depends on the diameter of the viewing lens. The larger the diameter better the image. Larger diameter instruments mean larger instrument channel and hence better irrigation using saline or water.

1. How to choose a nephroscope?

   A nephroscope can be chosen depending on the following features:

(a) Size:

Larger size nephroscopes

They have better vision due to larger sizes of lenses or larger diameter fibre bundles. They would also transmit better light due to obvious reason. A larger channel would also mean better continuous flow. Larger scopes are sturdier.

The prerequisite for use of larger scope is the use of a larger size of Amplatz sheath typically over 20 French. This allows good irrigation. This would allow easy clearance of blood clots and stone debris during the procedure. Better irrigation cools the operation site during ultrasonic lithotripsy.

The disadvantages include larger time for access and thus more exposure to radiation when using the image intensifier. The larger size of the Amplatz tract has also been correlated with an increased risk of bleeding.

The nomenclature for sizes varies as per various manufacturers and authors of various reports.

Conventional nephroscopes are available in sizes 24–32 Fr [1]. The scopes ranging from 14 to 22 Fr are known as MINI PCNL scopes. Sizes between 11 and 13 Fr are called ULTRA MINI [2]. The MICRO Perc system is 4.8 Fr in size [3].

(b) Scopes classified as per eye piece position

1. Offset eyepiece

   The Wickham type-The telescope makes an angle of 130° to the sheath

2. Amplatz type-The telescope is 90° to the sheath

   Rigid instruments and hand tools pass easily via the straight channel. The straight access sheath allows for the passage of rigid lithotripters and instruments. The irrigation channel ensures fluid flow. The fluid returns through the space between the nephroscope and its sheath. Hence the insertion of a large-diameter instruments results in reduction in flow.

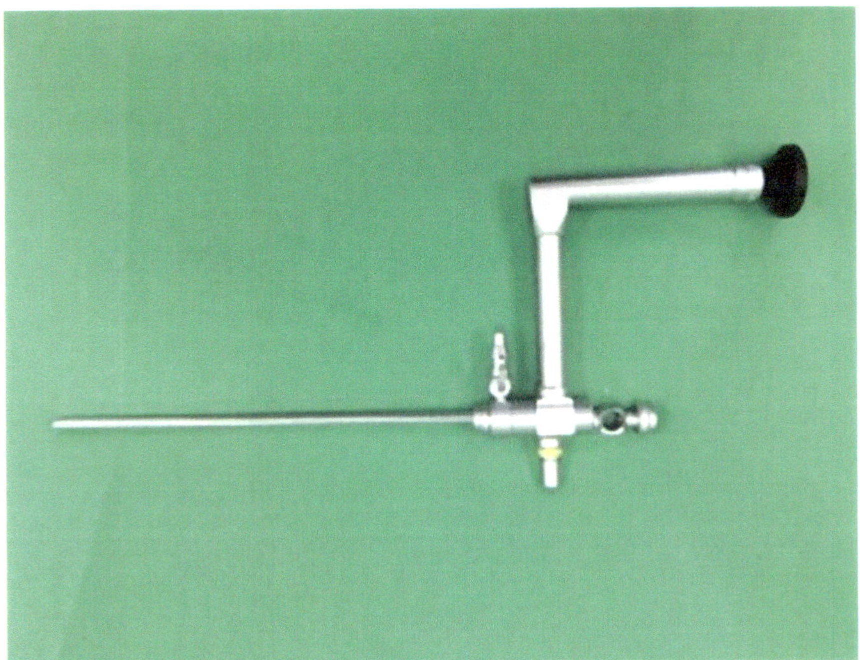

Fig. 6.1 Conventional rigid nephroscope showing eyepiece at right angle

The drawback of this system is noticed when nephroscope is torqued. This results in fragmented image and view distortion. The modern new systems use a hybrid design to avoid this issue (Fig. 6.1).

(c) Type of systems based on telescopes, i.e. 12°–30°.

(d) Depending on the length: standard length/long length—longer length scopes are used in obese patients, reaching intrarenal navigation to distant calyces or for operating bladder stones/morcellation. These would also mean using longer length Amplatz sheaths.

(e) The type of sheath-integrated scopes have a separate channel for flow and can be used without sheath.

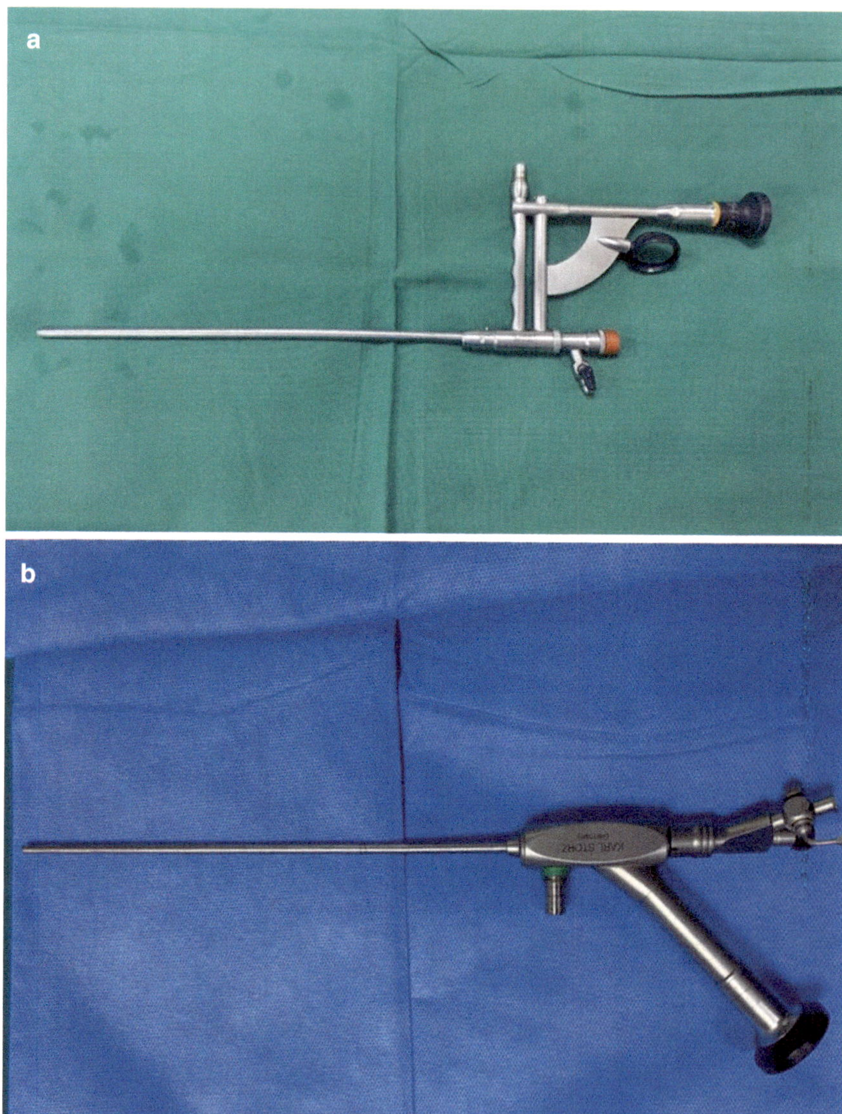

Fig. 6.2 (**a**) Shows conventional 20 Fr nephroscope. (**b**) MINISCOPE 12 Fr. Rigid nephroscope designs showing reducing sizes of endoscopes

The working channels of various scopes vary as per different manufacturers and they range from 10 to 12 Fr. The maximum size of instrument which can be passed from the instrument channel is 4–5 mm (Fig. 6.2a, b).

6.3 Methods of Sterilisation of Rigid Nephroscopes

All heat and vapour sensitive parts of the currently available endoscopes need effective sterilisation procedure so that critical procedures such as percutaneous renal surgery are guaranteed to be safe for the patient. This would reduce the sepsis chances and in turn avoid the burden of usage of higher antibiotics to treat infections related to the procedures.

Used nephroscopes are washed with high pressure water injection system and cleaned with enzyme solutions to free the channels of the blood and body fluid organic matter. These scopes are dried and subjected to one of the following methods of sterilisation.

Currently available nephroscopes are safe for autoclaving and we prefer to use Gamma sterilisation (Sterrad® Johnson & Johnson) for sterilisation.

6.3.1 Flexible Nephroscopes

Flexible scopes (see Fig. 6.3) use fibreoptic technology. It transmits the light in a nonlinear plane. Each scope uses three flexible fibreoptic bundles. Two bundles transmit light along with a solitary, glass imaging bundle. Each bundle is composed of thousands of fibres. The final image is a composite of images from individual fibres. Flexible endoscopes demonstrate deflections—the ability to flex in two directions at one or two positions. This is brought about by pulleys and cables which come from the tip. These are in turn attached to a working lever in the handle.

The operator rotates the handpiece and brings about movements in different planes. Though the fibres demonstrate excellent bendability, they are also prone to breakages. These result in the appearance of black dots or spots and will eventually lead to poor

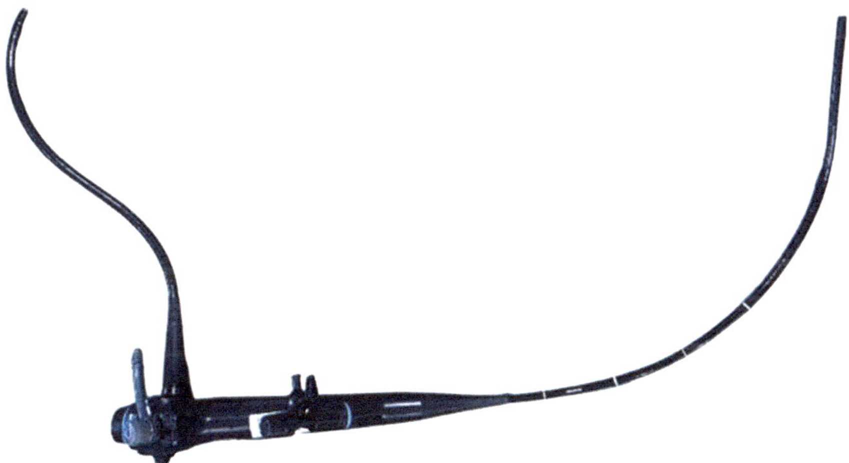

Fig. 6.3 Flexible fibreoptic cystonephroscope

vision due to poor light transmission. Typically, the damage to one fibre does not affect the image. However, many fractured fibres caused by wear on the scope do result in distortion of the final image. The working channels of flexible scopes allow simultaneous passage of fluid for irrigation and also the lithotripsy tools such as laser fibre or guide wires or stone baskets. The nephroscopes are typically 16 Fr in diameter with the maximum size of instruments which can be passed is 5 F [4] (Fig. 6.3).

6.4 Application and Use of Flexible Nephroscopes

Rigid scopes have no ability to enter small spaces such as calyces and can't bend inside the pelvicalyceal system. This is where flexible scopes with their nature to bend come in handy. They are able to take turns inside the system and look for the stones or fragments. They are useful for second look PCNL in cases of residual fragments. Application of 360 or 200 μm fibre using holmium laser results in dusting of stone fragments resulting in better stone-free rates [5].

The various studies published describing the stone-free rates do not have an agreement as to which is the size of residual fragments which is significant. Conventional X-rays typically detect about 5–6 mm fragments while ultrasound can detect at least 3 mm and CT KUB about 2 mm depending on the slice of CT [6]. The gold standard for residual fragment detection is however use of flexible scope during first or second look which does not miss much and is good to differentiate residual fragments from Randall's plaque.

6.5 Sterilisation of Flexible Scopes

These devices fall in category of treatment by minimally invasive surgery (MIS) where sterile instruments enter the body cavity and therapeutic or diagnostic procedures are carried out. These are regulated by FDA and would have to follow a process for cleaning and subsequent sterilisation not just disinfection.

Effective cleaning processes employed would need to eliminate all contamination including removal of biofilms. A method of checking for the leak would have been employed as per the manufacturers standard method. An effective drying would have to be done using pressurised air. A high-level disinfection procedure would involve chemical or gas sterilisation to ensure killing of all microorganisms. These however do not eliminate the spores [7].

Many studies have shown the superiority of terminal sterilisation using ethelene dioxide (ETO) and Gamma sterilisation as compared to chemical methods of sterilisation.

We recommend and use Sterrad® developed by Johnson & Johnson.

6.6 Newer Developments

6.6.1 Disposable Flexible Cystonephroscopes

Study recently published highlights the use of single use nephroscope as regards operator convenience, vision quality and stone-free status as well as safety of Ambuscope (Ambu R a scope)™ [4]. The study shows significant benefit in the user friendliness, ease of handling and last but not the least cost benefit—135 STERLING POUNDS VS 166 per use per patient. Similar cost benefit analysis done in other unit shows significant savings over a 90-day trial period indicating the future trend [8, 9].

References

1. Mulţescu R, Georgescu D, Geavlete PA, Geavlete B. Chapter 2—Equipment and instruments in percutaneous nephrolithotomy. In: Geavlete PA, editor. Percutaneous surgery of the upper urinary tract. New York: Academic Press; 2016. p. 3–24. https://doi.org/10.1016/B978-0-12-802404-1.00002-5.
2. Agrawal MS, Agarwal K, Jindal T, Sharma M. Ultra-mini-percutaneous nephrolithotomy: a minimally-invasive option for percutaneous stone removal. Indian J Urol. 2016;32(2):132–6.
3. Desai M, Mishra S. 'Microperc' micro percutaneous nephrolithotomy: evidence to practice. Curr Opin Urol. 2012;22(2):134–8. https://doi.org/10.1097/MOU.0b013e32834fc3bb.
4. Sabnis RB, Bhattu A, Mohankumar V. Sterilization of endoscopic instruments. Curr Opin Urol. 2014;24(2):195–202.
5. Gücük A, Kemahlı E, Üyetürk U, Tuygun C, Yıldız M, Metin A. Routine flexible nephroscopy for percutaneous nephrolithotomy for renal stones with low density: a prospective, randomized study. J Urol. 2013;190(1):144–8.
6. Harraz AM, Osman Y, El-Nahas AR, Elsawy AA, Fakhreldin I, Mahmoud O, et al. Residual stones after percutaneous nephrolithotomy: comparison of intraoperative assessment and postoperative non-contrast computerized tomography. World J Urol. 2017;35(8):1241–6.
7. Agrawal MS, Mukhilesh R, Mishra DK. Flexible mini nephroscopy. In: Agrawal MS, Mishra DK, Somani B, editors. Minimally invasive percutaneous nephrolithotomy. Singapore: Springer; 2022. p. 235–7. https://doi.org/10.1007/978-981-16-6001-6_21.
8. Assmus MMA, Krambeck AE, Lee MS, Agarwal DK, Mellon M, Rivera ME, et al. Cost-effectiveness of 90-day single-use flexible cystoscope trial: single center micro-costing analysis and user satisfaction. Urology. 2022;167:61–6.
9. Olaitan O, Pinnamaraju P, Nemade H, Pai A. 339° Single use flexible scopes in percutaneous renal surgery. Br J Surg. 2022;109(Supplement_1):znac039.224.

PCNL: Lithotripsy Devices

7

Subodh R. Shivde

"The expectations of life depend on diligence; the mechanic that would perfect his work must first sharpen his tools"

—Confucius

7.1 History of Lithotripsy

Early urological interventions consisted of the treatment of diseases of the lower urinary tract. There are reports of painful urinary retentions which if left untreated would lead to long-drawn illnesses. Historically stone treatment consisted of 'cutting over the stone' and drainage options included the insertion of metallic devices and bougies in the bladder. Some of these procedures were blind and needed many sittings. Opening of the bladder was performed by ancient Hindu Greek Roman and Arab surgeons. The complication rates were high and some of the interventions caused fistulae, infections and even death [1, 2].

7.2 Contemporary Instrumentation for Lithotripsy

7.2.1 Scientific Basis and Design Principles

7.2.1.1 Pneumatic Devices

Principle of technology: use of ballistic force generated by ultrasonic waves.

S. R. Shivde (✉)
Department of Urology, Deenanath Mangeshkar Hospital and Research Centre, Pune, Maharashtra, India

S. R. Shivde (ed.), *Techniques in Percutaneous Renal Stone Surgery*, https://doi.org/10.1007/978-981-19-9418-0_7

The handpiece is activated by pressure waves. A solid probe connected to the hand piece delivers the shocks resulting in breaking of stones. Pressure generated is approximately 3 atm. Stone is struck by oscillating probe and fragmentation occurs. This device is suited for small and intermediate size stones. Denstedt et al. described a new tool Swiss Lithoclast in 1992 [3].

The new device has been in use since then and multiple modifications have been tested showing that the device is safe, effective. It does not generate excessive heat and causes minimum or no tissue trauma [4, 5]. This device is time tested and proven very good for hard stones. The probe sizes available are 0.8–3 mm. The smaller sizes more suited for miniature scopes and the larger for conventional large scopes with sizes between 28 and 30 Fr.

The drawback of these devices is that the stone fragments would need manual removal and hence add to the duration of surgery and also cause residual stones. Since the probes are rigid, they cannot be used with flexible scopes.

7.2.1.2 Ultrasonic Probes

Principle of technology: electric current application to piezoelectric or piezoceramic crystals producing ultrasonic waves.

The handpiece consists of piezoelectric crystals. An electric current is applied to this crystal to generate an ultrasonic wave. This wave transmits through a metallic probe. It gets converted to vibrational energy at the tip of the probe. The stones get fragmented by the resultant mechanical waves. For this technology to be efficient, the lithotripsy probe needs to be in contact with the stone. Since no shock waves are generated the technology is safe for use in percutaneous surgery [6]. An irrigation channel with suction allows simultaneous evacuation of fragments and stone dust. Water or saline irrigation helps the cooling of the probe and avoids the generation of excessive heat. This modality is ideal for use in Struvite or soft matrix stones. The available probe sizes are 2.5–6 Fr, and the larger sizes allow the design to have hollow lumen through which suction could be applied.

Overheating of the probe can lead to tissue thermal damage. Direct contact with the tissue can lead to mucosal oedema and can lead to perforation of delate pelvicalyceal system [7].

7.2.1.3 Dual Probes

These use a combination of ballistic and ultrasonic technologies in a single probe. Both these tools could be used separately or in combination. The ultrasound device has suction attached to it. In combination mode, the pneumatic probe is passed through the ultrasonic probe. An attachment delivers compressed air for the pneumatic tool. A single pulse or combination mode delivers a frequency of 2–12 Hz. The ultrasonic device operates between 24 and 26 kHz. The higher frequencies are better suited for harder stones with chemical compositions consisting of calcium oxalate monohydrate, cysteine or calcium phosphate. The combination of devices results in faster clearing of stones in comparison to use of isolated technologies with similar rates of complications [8].

Practical Tip
To increase the speed of stone clearance first use dual modality and then remove pneumatic and apply ultrasonic with suction device. This trick would be ideally suited for large volume stones and staghorn stones.

7.2.1.4 Cyber Wand (Dual Probe Single Technology)

This technology uses dual probe ultrasound. The small probe (21 kHz) is fixed to the hand piece and the longer outer probe is connected via a free mass in hand piece (1000 Hz). This being slow has a ballistic effect. The inner probe has 2.1 mm lumen, and outer probe has a diameter of 3.75 mm. The smaller lumen leads to limited suction and hence limits rapid stone clearance. This necessitates use of additional extraction devices at the end of procedure [9].

7.2.1.5 Shock Pulse (Shock Pulse SE Olympus) (Single Probe Dual Modality)

This device has both ultrasonic and ballistic mechanism in single probe. The device consists of hand piece and a foot pedal. The piezoelectric crystal in the hand piece produces 21 kHz waves in the vibrating phase. Free mass elements are incorporated in the hand piece. The proximal end of which oscillates to produce mechanical waves. Waves are then transmitted to a spring which causes the probe to vibrate. The frequency of oscillation is 300 Hz. This produces the desired ballistic effect. The suction can be adjusted by a dial on the hand piece. The available probe sizes are 2.91–3.76 Fr. In a comparative study using the Cyberwand, Lithoclast Master and ultrasonic device, Chew et al. found the shock pulse device more efficient with faster fragmentation and rapid evacuation of fragments [10].

7.2.1.6 Swiss Lithoclast Trilogy

This new device uses ultrasound and ballistic technology. There is a traditional foot pedal, and the hand device does not have any controls. Available probe sizes are 3–11.7 Fr. Carlos et al. compared the single probe dual energy models trilogy and shock pulse with traditional ultrasonic device in an in vitro stone model. They found that the trilogy was much faster to deliver results and had better clearance rates [11].

7.2.1.7 Holmium YAG (Ho:YAG) Laser

This works with photothermal effect. The wavelength 2140 nm is highly absorbed in water leading to a wide margin of safety. The wattage ranges are 10–80 W with higher range application more suited for tissue applications such as tissue cutting, prostate enucleation and stricture cutting (laser VIU). The pulse duration can be increased to reduce stone retropulsion. The stone remains stable during long pulse leading to less chasing. This also leads to less fibre tip degradation also known as Burn Back.

Pulse modulation—the initial pulse causes the vaporisation of fluid between the fibre tip and target, i.e. stone and the second pulse follows and travels through vapour channel before hitting the target. This leads to stable stone fragments and reduced retropulsion with increased fragmentation. The Lumenis Moses Pulse™ 120 W with short medium and long pulse durations with modulation mode. This device has 2 modes: distance and contact. This system is an example of closed platform laser with no adaptability to use fibres made by other parties. The Olympus EMPOWER™ available in 35 W, 65 W, 100 W uses the stabilisation mode similar to above-mentioned pulse modulation.

Laser Fibres

These are made of low hydroxy silica optic fibres to transfer energy between console and target. The fibres available range from 150 to 1000 μm flexible scopes allow the use of 150–300 μm fibres. The 300–365 μm fibres are used with MINI Perc systems and conventional nephoscopes.

7.2.1.8 Thulium Fibre Laser (TFL)

This is a relatively new technology. The conventional YAG crystal is an ion doped crystal. TFL uses a fibre which is thulium doped. This diode laser channels energy via the fibre. This leads to electron activation which in turn leads to activation of photons. The resultant energy is made to reach the surgical site using a fibre.

Enikeev et al. using Thulium Fibre Laser (NTO IRE-Polus Russia) reported 85% stone free rates using 0.8 Joules (25–30 W) with a frequency of 31–38 Hz. They reported a retropulsion rate of 17% and less than 3% rate of poor visibility in this study where 153 patients enrolled for the study [12]. In another study by Mahajan et al. they compared holmium laser lithotripsy with thulium fibre laser for cases undergoing MINI Perc (Miniaturised Percutaneous Lithotripsy) [13].

They reported 94.9% stone free rates for TFL versus 90.9% for holmium laser lithotripsy.

The TFL group however had a self-limiting post operative haematuria of unexplained origin which did not need any intervention.

References

1. Bloom DA. Hippocrates and urology: the first surgical subspecialty. Urology. 1997;50(1):157–9.
2. Trompoukis C, Giannakopoulos S, Touloupidis S. Lithotomy by empirical doctors in the 19th century: a traditional surgical technique that lasted through the centuries. J Urol. 2007;178(6):2284–6.
3. Denstedt JD, Eberwein PM, Singh RR. The Swiss Lithoclast: a new device for intracorporeal lithotripsy. J Urol. 1992;148(3, Part 2):1088–90.
4. Patel SR, Nakada SY. The modern history and evolution of percutaneous nephrolithotomy. J Endourol. 2015;29(2):153–7.
5. Wollin DA, Lipkin ME. Emerging technologies in ultrasonic and pneumatic lithotripsy. Urol Clin. 2019;46(2):207–13.
6. Knudsen BE. Instrumentation for stone disease. In: Best SL, Nakada SY, editors. Minimally invasive urology: an essential clinical guide to endourology, laparoscopy, LESS and robotics. Cham: Springer International Publishing; 2020. p. 169–93. https://doi.org/10.1007/978-3-030-23993-0_11.
7. Monga M, Rane A. Percutaneous renal surgery. New York: Wiley; 2014. p. 312.

8. Lehman DS, Hruby GW, Phillips C, Venkatesh R, Best S, Monga M, et al. Prospective randomized comparison of a combined ultrasonic and pneumatic lithotrite with a standard ultrasonic lithotrite for percutaneous nephrolithotomy. J Endourol. 2008;22(2):285–90.
9. York NE, Borofsky MS, Chew BH, Dauw CA, Paterson RF, Denstedt JD, et al. Randomized controlled trial comparing three different modalities of lithotrites for intracorporeal lithotripsy in percutaneous nephrolithotomy. J Endourol. 2017;31(11):1145–51.
10. Scotland KB, Kroczak T, Pace KT, Chew BH. Stone technology: intracorporeal lithotripters. World J Urol. 2017;35(9):1347–51.
11. Carlos EC, Wollin DA, Winship BB, Jiang R, Radvak D, Chew BH, et al. In vitro comparison of a novel single probe dual-energy lithotripter to current devices. J Endourol. 2018;32(6):534–40.
12. Enikeev D, Taratkin M, Klimov R, Alyaev Y, Rapoport L, Gazimiev M, et al. Thulium-fiber laser for lithotripsy: first clinical experience in percutaneous nephrolithotomy. World J Urol. 2020;38(12):3069–74.
13. Mahajan AD, Mahajan SA. Thulium fiber laser versus holmium: yttrium aluminium garnet laser for stone lithotripsy during mini-percutaneous nephrolithotomy: a prospective randomized trial. Indian J Urol. 2022;38(1):42–7.

8 PCNL Accessories: Guide Wires and Baskets

Subodh R. Shivde

8.1 Historical Aspects

Sven Ivar Seldinger (1921–1998) a radiologist at Karolinska institute in Sweden first performed the procedure to enter the lumen of vessel. This is popularly known as Seldinger technique. He demonstrated the fact that it is safer than a blind procedure. This procedure involves puncturing the structure, then a passage of guide wire. The needle is then removed and dilator is passed. The needle is removed and dilator is passed. The dilator is removed and the catheter is passed [1].

An ideal guide wire is

(a) Cheap, readily available, easy to sterilize
(b) Light and easy to handle
(c) Strong to avoid easy bending
(d) Resist stripping easily in case of coated wires
(e) Atraumatic and easy to manoeuvre
(f) No systemic effects

The use of guide wires allows an endourologist to navigate through the pelvicalyceal system and also a safe passage for instrument navigation. The currently available guide wires in common use are 0.035, 0.038 and 0.025 inches. They have variable lengths such as 140 or 150 cm. These typically have an inner steel core and an out smooth coating. Flexible tip ready focus wire M (Terumo™) or Sensor Dual Flex (Boston Scientific™) are available. They are least likely to perforate and show the lowest withdrawal force and possess good memory [2, 3].

S. R. Shivde (✉)
Department of Urology, Deenanath Mangeshkar Hospital and Research Centre, Pune, Maharashtra, India

S. R. Shivde (ed.), *Techniques in Percutaneous Renal Stone Surgery*, https://doi.org/10.1007/978-981-19-9418-0_8

8.2 Structure and Design of the Currently Available Guide Wires

8.2.1 Steel Guide Wires

These are cheap and strong in structure with easy torqueability. They do not deform easily and hence can cause organ damage in case of abnormal placement. Amplatz Super stiff™ is an example of such wires by Boston Scientific.

8.2.2 Alloy-Based Guide Wires

These are made with nickel and titanium popularly known as NITINOL wires. These are lighter and more flexible. J tip wires tend to bend easily and hence are less 'Pushable' (Fig. 8.2). The flexibility allows negotiation of spaces such as pelvic cavity, ureters and pelviureteric junctions.

8.2.3 Hydrophilic Guide Wires

These are steel or nitinol core wires which are coated with polytetrafluoroethylene (PTFE) or silicone. These coatings reduce coefficient of friction and allow an easy passage during procedure. They however tend to very slippery and loss of access is seen when they slip out accidentally. They are coated to half their length and need to be wet before use [4].

8.2.4 Guide Wires—Which and When

Hydrophilic wires are commonly used for smooth passage through narrow areas. They are used to get out of difficulties. PTFE and silicone coatings reduce coefficient of friction (Figs. 8.1 and 8.2).

The stiffer wires (Zebra) and steel core wires are good for passage of stents and catheters as they resist bending giving more firmness to the operator (Fig. 8.3).

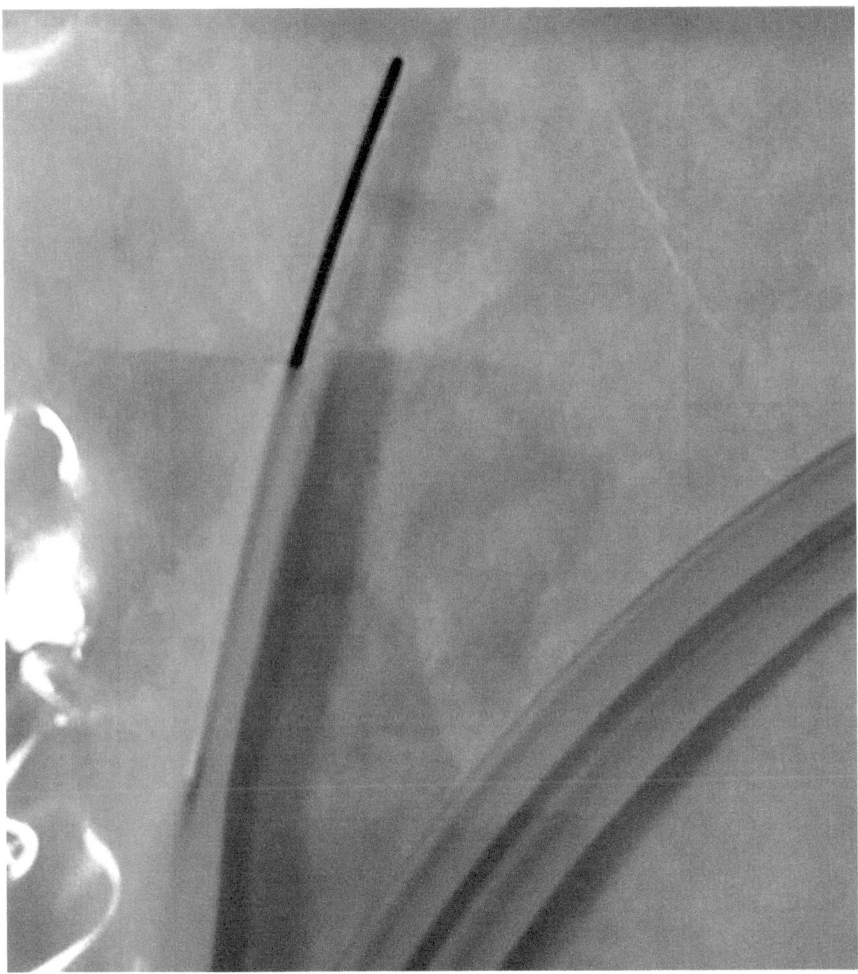

Fig. 8.1 Straight tip guide wire

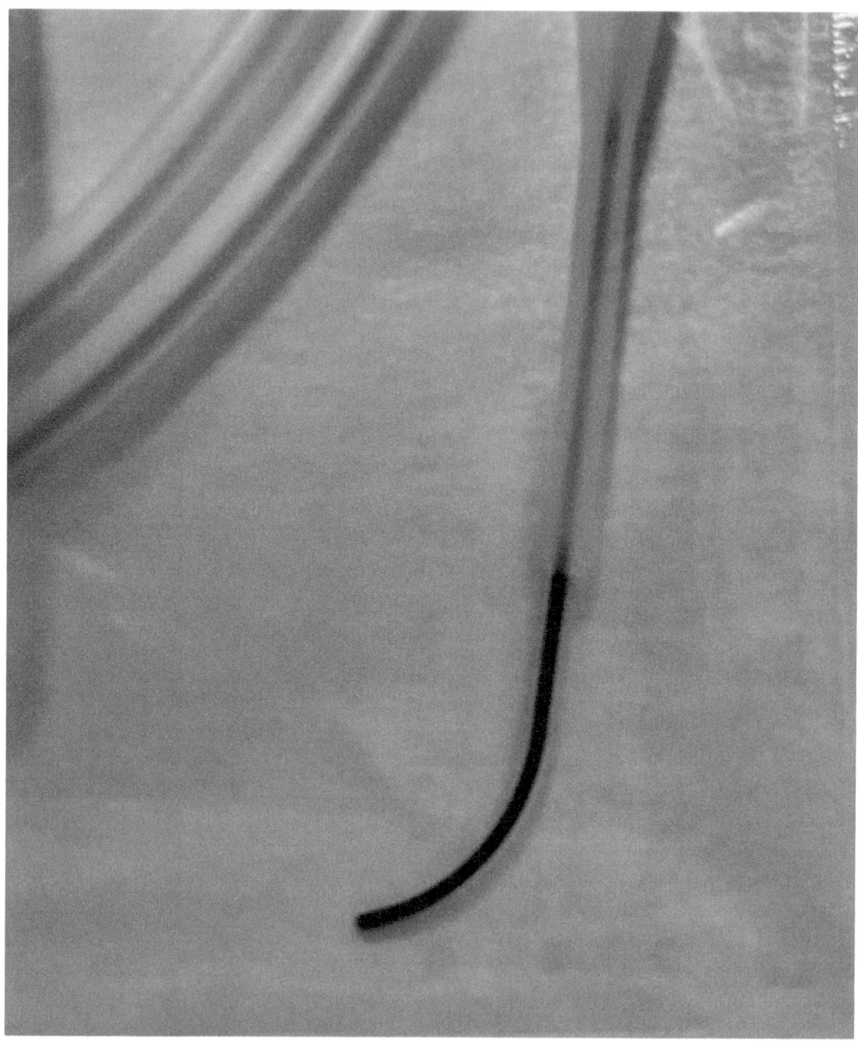

Fig. 8.2 J tip guide wire

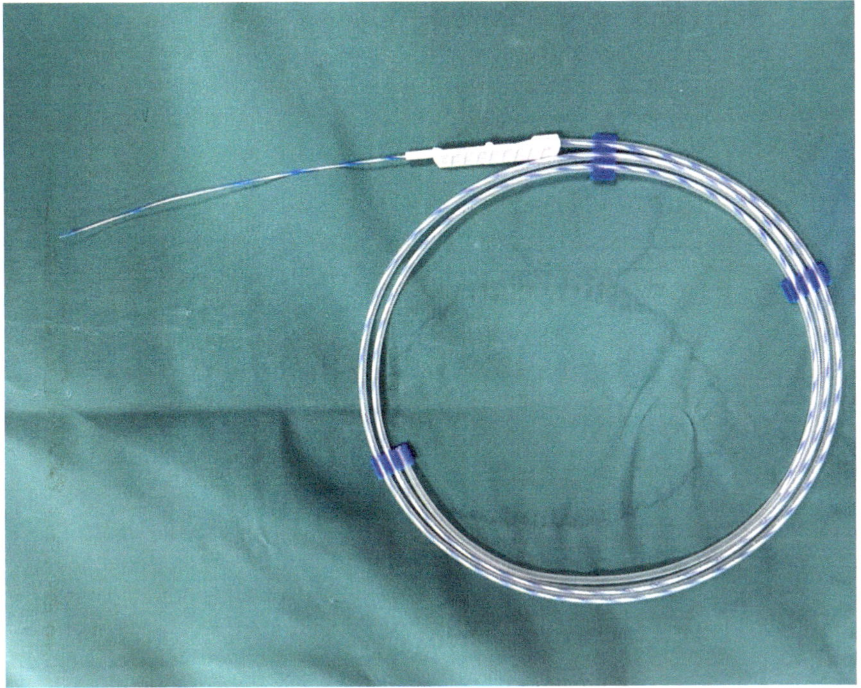

Fig. 8.3 Zebra wire

8.3 Guide Wire Complications

If it can happen it will—Anon

Local complications

(a) Local injury, tissue dissection and rupture of delicate pelvicalyceal system. Remedy: Early recognition, stop the procedure and use image intensifier continuously to monitor the progress of passage of instruments.
(b) Vessel injury: entry in major vessel causing bleeding.
(c) Sepsis.
(d) Shearing of wire: recognize early, re-insert a new wire, look for pieces of coating and retrieve with forceps. Unrecognized pieces retained in the kidney will lead to formation of kidney stones. This situation is also a potential for medicolegal liability.
(e) Knotting of wires: looping of a wire is a precursor to knotting [5]. If a knot forms use a tract dilator over the outer free portion of the wire to tighten the knot and then pull out the wire in entirety. Mosseri et al. reported a 'Straight Wire' sign for early extrusion, e.g. guide wire during percutaneous coronary surgery. Identification of abnormal path of the wire should be picked up by experienced urologist or assisting persons to avoid further damage [6].

8.3.1 Holmium Lasers and Guide Wires

Holmium laser could easily cut the wire in the passage during lithotripsy. Abrasions caused due to firing of lasers would result in difficulties in passage of stents over these wires. It is prudent to change such wire and replace it with a better wire.

8.3.2 Stone Retrieval Devices (Baskets and Forceps)

It is necessary to retrieve all seen fragments from the pelvicalyceal system after a good stone disintegration. Stone particles are needed for biochemical examination, and a good stone clearance means better outcomes. Traditionally the Dormia spiral stone baskets have been used for clearance of ureteral stone fragments [7]. Originally described and used for ureteral stones and retrieval, these have found wide range of applications in gastroenterological field.

They are however not without their problems such as mechanical malfunction, impaction in situ with stone embedded within and damage to the urothelium causing perforations and formation of urinoma and eventually sepsis. Strictures have been reported as long-term complications of use of baskets and retrieval devices [8]. Stone held in open jaw of the retrieval forceps would lead to size disparity between the forceps and channel of nephroscope, making removal through the channel difficult. In such a case it is advised to drop the stone back, come out with the forceps and nephroscope assembly and re-enter (Fig. 8.4a, b).

Baskets and other devices for this purpose have been undergoing rapid changes in design and structure to get an optimum output without compromising the safety of patients. Traditionally stainless steel has been used which is strong but hard to cut if stone embedding occurs. We could thus think of use of holmium laser if such a need arises [9]. NITINOL baskets have been popular since the material is soft and pliable with memory which increases the safety and is virtually atraumatic to the renal papilla. The Tipless NITINOL baskets have been very useful for this purpose (Fig. 8.5a, b).

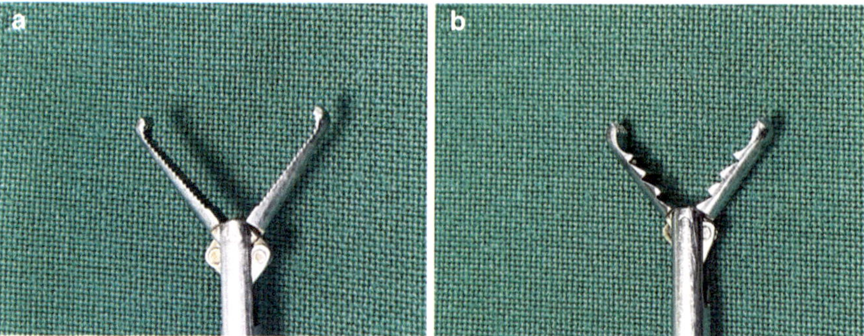

Fig. 8.4 (**a**) Showing straight blades. (**b**) Showing 'crocodile jaw' type of forceps. (**a**, **b**) 2 Types of stone retrieval forceps differing in jaw shapes

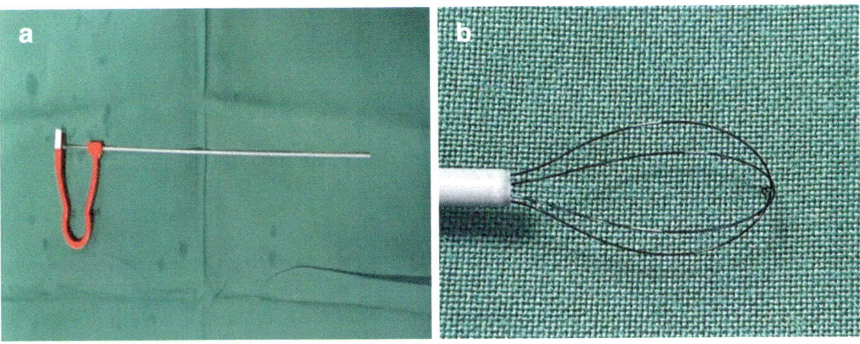

Fig. 8.5 (**a**) PERC NGage nitinol stone basket (COOK™). (**b**) Close up view of open basket—note the tipless atraumatic design

Honey published a comparative study in pig model kidneys with three operators using the 3.2 Fr Nitinol Tipless baskets versus 3 Fr flat wire baskets. They concluded that the nitinol tipless allowed bending of scopes for better visualization with minimum procedure time and very little trauma [10].

References

1. Kipling M, Mohammed A, Medding RN. Guidewires in clinical practice: applications and troubleshooting. Expert Rev Med Devices. 2009;6(2):187–95.
2. Liguori G, Antoniolli F, Trombetta C, Biasotto M, Amodeo A, Pomara G, et al. Comparative experimental evaluation of guidewire use in urology. Urology. 2008;72(2):286–9.
3. Hinck BD, Emmott AS, Omar M, Tarplin S, Chew BH, Monga M. Hybrid guidewires: analysis and comparison of the mechanical properties and safety profiles. Can Urol Assoc J. 2019;13(2):59–63. https://cuaj.ca/index.php/journal/article/view/5396
4. Torricelli FCM, De S, Sarkissian C, Monga M. Hydrophilic guidewires: evaluation and comparison of their properties and safety. Urology. 2013;82(5):1182–6.
5. Joshi PM, Shivde SR, Dighe TA. Knotting of the guide wires: a rare complication during minimally invasive procedure on kidney-lessons learnt. J Minim Access Surg. 2008;4(4):114–6.
6. Mosseri M, Banai S, Jabara R, Rott D. The straight wire sign: recognizing guidewire exit during percutaneous coronary intervention for chronic total occlusion. Int J Cardiol. 2007;116(3):e106–8.
7. Dormia E. Dormia basket: standard technique, observations, and general concepts. Urology. 1982;20(4):437.
8. de la Rosette JJ, Skrekas T, Segura JW. Handling and prevention of complications in stone basketing. Eur Urol. 2006;50(5):991–8. https://doi.org/10.1016/j.eururo.2006.02.033.
9. Teichman JM, Kamerer AD. Use of the holmium: YAG laser for the impacted stone basket. J Urol. 2000;164(5):1602–3.
10. Honey RJ. Assessment of a new tipless nitinol stone basket and comparison with an existing flat-wire basket. J Endourol. 1998;12(6):529–31.

9 PCNL: Small to Smaller: A Journey from Max to Mini to Micro

Small to Very Small Scopes in PCNL: Does Size Matters?

Ravindra Sabnis and V. Mohankumar

9.1 Introduction

Percutaneous nephrolithotomy (PCNL) is the procedure of choice for treatment of renal calculi. Since it was described in the eighties, it has undergone evolution with regard to choice of access, method of dilatation, and the energy source used for fragmentation of the stone. The indications have changed over the years with the introduction of other techniques such as extracorporeal shockwave lithotripsy (ESWL) and flexible ureterorenoscopy. In last two decades, PCNL instruments have also undergone miniaturization with introduction of Miniperc™, Ultraminiperc™, Microperc™. Question remains whether this small to very small size of PCNL tract is worth it? What are the advantages? Whether this reduction in tract size has made any difference in success rate and safety aspects of PCNL. In this chapter, we shall discuss all such aspects and rationality of small tract size in percutaneous renal surgery for stones.

9.2 History of PCNL

The first percutaneous nephrostomy description of record was published in 1865 by Thomas Hillier [1]. However in 1976, Fernström and Johansson [2] were the first to describe a technique for extracting renal calculi through a percutaneous nephrostomy under radiological control. Technique was further refined and described by Peter Alken and Arthur Smith in 1979. This marks the beginning of PCNL era. PCNL during those days was done with large size tract—40–42 F and often intact removal of stone. Larger stone removal was possible with invention of energy sources to disintegrate the stone, introduction of specially designed nephroscopes

R. Sabnis (✉) · V. Mohankumar
Department of Urology, Muljibhai Patel Urological Hospital, Nadiad, Gujarat, India

S. R. Shivde (ed.), *Techniques in Percutaneous Renal Stone Surgery*, https://doi.org/10.1007/978-981-19-9418-0_9

and forceps to remove fragments. However, in early eighties, complications rates were very high especially bleeding complications. Hence PCNL was contraindicated in solitary kidney, pediatric patients, staghorn stones, anomalous (horseshoe, ectopic) kidney stones. Fear was of bleeding complications which may result in kidney loss. Extensive studies, data analysis suggested that tract size may be responsible for complications.

9.3 Does Tract Size Matters?

Does it really matter what tract of PCNL you choose? Will it reduce the complication rate? Will it affect success—clearance rate? These aspects are extensively studied in the last two decades. Common complications of PCNL are bleeding—intraoperative or postoperative, perforation, calyceal tear, infundibular tear, damage to surrounding structures, persistent leak, pain, and nephron loss. CROES study [3] suggested that major complications of PCNL were bleeding (7.8%), perforation (3.4%), and hydrothorax (1.8%).

The bleeding complications can be attributed to the tract size. CROES study [3] states that the sheath size is an important predictor of bleeding complications. Kukreja et al. [4] have also proven that reducing the tract size reduces the incidence of bleeding especially in pediatric patients. Mishra et al. [5] have also mentioned that reduction in tract size reduces bleeding and the hospital stay while maintaining similar clearance rates. Bhattu et al. [6] had observed that access via multiple tracts does not result in significant blood loss if the tract size was less. Cheng et al. [7] have also observed that reducing tract size results in less bleeding without affecting the clearance rates.

Pain can also be attributed to tract size. Knoll et al. [8] had confirmed that reduction in tract size results in less pain and decrease in postoperative analgesic requirement. Desai et al. [9] had observed that pain was maximum with large sized nephrostomy.

Monga et al. [10] concluded that reduction in tract size reduces the volume of renal parenchyma that is dilated and thereby causes reduction in postoperative pain, bleeding and scarring. Guven et al. [11] concluded that reduction in tract size reduces bleeding in pediatric population and hence recommended Miniperc in children. Thus, there is ample evidence in literature to support that tract size is directly proportional to complications.

9.4 Era of Miniaturization

It is obvious that if tract size is less, complications will be less. Hence all research in PCNL in last two decades revolved around reducing tract size. Enormous research in energy sources to break the stones is key factor in introducing small size nephroscopes. Initially ultrasonic energy was the commonest energy source to break the stones. Other energy sources like EHL did not stand the test of time. Ultrasonic probes could not be too small and hence for many years, nephroscope sizes varied from 24 to 28 F. However, when pneumatic energy was introduced, which was equally powerful to break the stones, reduction of tract size was further possible. Smallest probe of pneumatic lithotripter was as small as 0.8 mm. Introduction of holmium laser triggered further reduction in size of nephroscope. Fiber size now available is as small as 200 μm. This made emergence of variety of procedures like Miniperc, Ultraminiperc, Microperc, Minimicroperc. This marked the beginning of the era of minimally invasive PCNL.

Miniperc is PCNL done with sheath size less than or equal to 20 Fr. The term was coined by Jackman et al. [12] who defined it as percutaneous nephrolithotomy achieved through a sheath too small to accommodate standard rigid nephoscope. Miniperc was originally devised for handling stones in children by Helal et al. [13] who devised the peel away sheath for Miniperc. In the year 2000, Negle devised the Miniperc Storz system. Miniperc has been widely used in adults because of its ability to minimize blood loss and hasten recovery and with similar clearance rates. In Miniperc, the scopes used range from 12 to 14 Fr, and the tract size varies from 15 to 20 Fr. Both Lithoclast™ and laser can be used for stone breaking modalities in mini PCNL. Mini PCNL can also be used in situations where the infundibulum is narrow and the smaller size of the scope can be used to navigate through the narrow infundibulum. Miniperc is ideally suited for treating stones of sizes varying from 1 to 2.5 cm. However, several centers are removing large bulk and staghorn stones by Miniperc [14–16]. Lahme et al. [14] proved that Miniperc is efficient in clearance of large bulk stones with good success rate. Sung et al. [16] have achieved a stone free rate of 95% in stones of size less than 6 cm. Another advantage of Miniperc in large stones is to utilize it for accessary tracts. When major portion of large stone with multiple calyceal stones or staghorn stones is removed with standard PCNL, for inaccessible stones, accessary tracts can be made with use of Miniperc technique. This will significantly reduce complications of multiple tract PCNLs.

In a prospective study, Mishra et al. [5] proved that Miniperc has equal efficiency in clearing stones, as compared to standard PCNL for stones less than 2 cm. Biggest advantages were significantly less hemoglobin drop and making the procedures tubeless. However, procedure time was significantly higher. Probably because of reduced visibility, non-clearing of small clots hampering the vision and need to reduce the fragments to a much smaller size.

In small stones, RIRS is also a modality of choice [17, 18]. Sabnis et al. [17] compared RIRS and Miniperc for stones <2 cm size and found that Miniperc has significantly less operative time and higher clearance rate. Miniperc also avoids need of DJ stents in majority of cases thereby reducing all the problems related to DJ stents. However, Miniperc has more Hb drop as compared to RIRS.

In 2013, Desai et al. [19] introduced the technique of U*ltraminiperk* which further reduced the tract size. The authors dilated the tract up to 11–13 Fr and achieved stone fragmentation using 365-μ holmium laser fiber under direct vision of the 3.5 Fr ultra-thin telescope and the fragment retrieval being done using a specially designed sheath by creating an eddy current of saline.

A step further in miniaturization was the application of the "all seeing needle" of Microperc by Desai et al. [20]. Microperc uses 16 G needle. Authors feel ideal indication for Microperc is stone <1.5 cm and puncture should be directly on the stone. Several centers have adopted this modality and compared the technique with RIRS [21]. Main advantage of Microperc is ability to treat stones in the lower calyx or in any other calyx which is situated at an awkward angle and hence difficult to access by flexible ureterorenoscope (URS). The potential disadvantage of this method is possibility of developing high intrarenal pressures and inability to retrieve fragments after disintegration. Microperc is used to treat stones in pediatric population with good results [22].

9.5 Uniformity in Nomenclature

As tract size of PCNL was going down, several authors coined their own terminology like Miniperc, minimally invasive PNL, Ultraminiperc, Microperc, Minimicroperc, etc. To develop uniformity, Schilling et al. [23] suggested uniform nomenclature, which gives clear idea about which size tract is being used. It is proposed that tract size should be described as in Table 9.1.

Storz adopted this nomenclature and their new generation MIP system is as per this nomenclature. Telescope of 19.5 F to be used with 23/24 and 25/26 sheaths. Telescope of 12 F to be used with 15/16, 16.5/17.5 and 21/22 F sheaths. Telescope of 7.5 F to be used with 11/12 and 8.5/9.5 sheaths. When these sheaths are used with respective telescope—it is supposed to create a vacuum cleaner effect based on venture principle and Bernoulli effect [24]. With vacuum cleaner effect, a pseudo-bubble is created which traps small fragment and as telescope is withdrawn, fragment move along with it and eventually drops out of sheath. This obviates the need to use any forceps for fragment extraction.

Table 9.1 PCN tract sizes

Description	Tract size
XL	≥25 Fr
L	20 to <25 Fr
M	15 to <20 Fr
S	10 to <15 Fr
XS	5 to <10 Fr
XXS	<5 Fr

9.6 MIP in Relation to SWL, RIRS

Majority of patients now present with small renal stones probably because increased health awareness, routine health checkups, easy availability of detection modalities like ultrasound. Hence all modalities like SWL, RIRS to treat such stones have to be compared with MIP. Even SWL is becoming refined with better shock wave generators. Slender digital FURS gives excellent vision with ability to reach each calyx. Thinner laser fibers of 200 μ does not compromise deflection of FURS. Although guidelines still suggest SWL as method of choice for stones <10 mm, treatment has to be individualized depending upon expertise of surgeon, availability of instruments… etc. All these modalities are extensively compared in literature claiming some advantages and disadvantages to all modalities of treatment [21, 25–27].

9.7 Conclusion

Small tract size PCNL certainly has many advantages. However how small is ideal is not yet clear. As smaller and smaller tract is used, 9.5 or 4.85 F, fragment extraction and procedure time, become a big concern. Although as of today, Miniperc still remains good modality, prospective studies will clarify, how small can we go further and whether it is worth it.

References

1. Nour H, Kamal A, Ghobashi S, et al. Percutaneous nephrolithotomy in the supine position: safety and outcomes in a single-centre experience. Arab J Urol. 2013;11:62–7.
2. Ferstrom I, Johansson B. Percutaneous pyelolithotomy: a new extraction technique. Scand J Urol Nephrol. 1976;10:257–9.
3. de la Rosette J, Assimos D, Desai M, et al. The Clinical Research Office of the Endourological Society Percutaneous Nephrolithotomy Global Study: indications, complications, and outcomes in 5803 patients. J Endourol. 2011;25:11–7.
4. Kukreja R, Desai M, Patel S, Bapat S, Desai M. First prize: factors affecting blood loss during percutaneous nephrolithotomy: prospective study. J Endourol. 2004;18(8):715–22.
5. Mishra S, Sharma R, Garg C, Kurien A, Sabnis R, Desai M. Prospective comparative study of Miniperc and standard PNL for treatment of 1–2 cm size renal stone. BJU Int. 2011;108(6):896–9.
6. Bhattu AS, Mishra S, Ganpule A, Jagtap J, Vijaykumar M, Sabnis RB, Desai M. Outcomes in a large series of Minipercs: analysis of consecutive 318 patients. J Endourol. 2014;29(3):283–7.
7. Cheng F, Yu W, Zhang X, et al. Minimally invasive tract in percutaneous nephrolithotomy for renal stones. J Endourol. 2010;24:1579–82.
8. Knoll T, Wezel F, Michel MS, et al. Do patients benefit from miniaturized tubeless percutaneous nephrolithotomy? A comparative prospective study. J Endourol. 2010;24:1075–9.
9. De Sio M, Autorino R, Quattrone. Choosing the nephrosotmy suize after percutaneous nephrolithotomy. World J Urol. 2011;29:707–11.

10. Monga M, Oglevie S. Minipercutaneous nephrolithotomy. J Endourol. 2000;14:419–21.
11. Guven S, Istanbulluoglu O, Ozturk A, et al. Percutaneous nephrolithotomy is highly efficient and safe in infants and children under 3 years of age. Urol Int. 2010;85:455–60.
12. Jackman SV, Hedican SP, Peters CA, Docimo SG. Percutaneous nephrolithotomy in infants and preschool age children: experience with a new technique. Urology. 1998;52:697–701.
13. Helal M, Black T, Lockhart J, Figueroa TE. The Hickman peel away sheath: alternative to pediatric nephrolithotomy. J Endourol. 1997;11:171–2.
14. Lahme S, Bichler KH, Strohmaier WL, Götz T. Minimally invasive PCNL in patients with renal pelvic and calyceal stones. Eur Urol. 2001;40(6):619–24.
15. Wong C, Leveillee RJ. Single upper pole percutaneous access for treatment of ≥5 cm complex branched staghorn calculi. J Endourol. 2002;16:477–81.
16. Sung YM, Choo SW, Jeon SS, et al. The "mini-perc" technique of percutaneous nephrolithotomy with a 14-Fr peel-away sheath: 3-year results in 72 patients. Korean J Radiol. 2006;7(1):50–6.
17. Sabnis RB, Jagtap J, Mishra S, Desai M. Treating renal calculi 1–2 cm in diameter with minipercutaneous or retrograde intrarenal surgery: a prospective comparative study. BJU Int. 2012;110:E346–9.
18. Sofer M, Watterson JD, Wollin TA, Nott L, Razvi H, Denstedt JD. Holmium:YAG laser lithotripsy for upper urinary tract calculi in 598 patients. J Urol. 2002;167:31–4.
19. Desai JD, Zeng G, Zhao Z, et al. A novel technique of ultra-mini-percutaneous nephrolithotomy: introduction and an initial experience for treatment of upper urinary calculi less than 2 cm. Biomed Res Int. 2013;2013:490793.
20. Desai MR, Sharma R, Mishra S, et al. Single-step percutaneous nephrolithotomy (microperc): the initial clinical report. J Urol. 2011;186:140–5.
21. Sabnis RB, Ganesamoni R, Doshi A, Ganpule AP, Jagtap J, Desai MR. Micropercutaneous nephrolithotomy (microperc) vs retrograde intrarenal surgery for the management of small renal calculi: a randomized controlled trial. BJU Int. 2013;112(3):355–61.
22. Silay MS, Tepeler A, Atis G, Sancaktutar AA, Piskin M, Gurbuz C, Penbegul N, Ozturk A, Caskurlu T, Armagan A. Initial report of microperc in the treatment of pediatric nephrolithiasis. J Pediatr Surg. 2013;48(7):1578–83.
23. Schilling D, Hüsch T, Bader M, Herrmann TR, Nagele U. Nomenclature in PCNL or the tower of babel: a proposal for a uniform terminology. World J Urol. 2015;33(11):1905–7. https://doi.org/10.1007/s00345-015-1506-7.
24. Nicklas AP, Schilling D, Bader MJ, Herrmann TR, Nagele U. The vacuum cleaner effect in minimally invasive percutaneous nephrolitholapaxy. World J Urol. 2015;33(11):1847–53.
25. Srisubat A, Potisat S, Lojanapiwat B, et al. Extracorporeal shock wave lithotripsy (ESWL) versus percutaneous nephrolithotomy (PCNL) or retrograde intrarenal surgery (RIRS) for kidney stones. Cochrane Database Syst Rev. 2009;7:CD00704.
26. Sahinkanat T, Ekerbicer H, Onal B, et al. Evaluation of the effects of relationships between main spatial lower pole calyceal anatomic factors on the success of shock-wave lithotripsy in patients with lower pole kidney stones. Urology. 2008;71(5):801–5.
27. Danuser H, Muller R, Descoeudres B, et al. Extracorporeal shock wave lithotripsy of lower calyx calculi: how much is treatment outcome influenced by the anatomy of the collecting system? Eur Urol. 2007;52(2):539–46.

"MICRO-PERC": A Journey from Small to Very Small

10

Arvind P. Ganpule, Jaspreet Singh Chabra, and Mahesh R. Desai

Abbreviations

Ho-YAG	Holmium-yttrium aluminum garnet
MeSH	Medical subject headings
PCNL	Percutaneous nephrolithotomy
RIRS	Retrograde intrarenal surgery
SWL	Shockwave lithotripsy

10.1 Introduction

We saw in the previous chapter the technique of miniaturization of the scopes and the resultant effects on it's efficacy and drawbacks. The use of laser especially the holmium laser with fibers ranging from 200 micron to 550 microns led to further improvisations and refinements in the miniaturization of the nephroscopes. The previously available standard nephroscopes were (>20 F) and the Miniperc (12–20 F) and the ultra mini-perc (11–13 F) (Figs. 10.1 and 10.2). We discuss the smallest scope available as a result of these refinements (16 G) (Fig. 10.3) also termed the Microperc.

A. P. Ganpule (✉) · J. S. Chabra · M. R. Desai
Muljibhai Patel Urological Hospital, Nadiad, Gujarat, India
e-mail: mrdesai@mpuh.org

S. R. Shivde (ed.), *Techniques in Percutaneous Renal Stone Surgery*,
https://doi.org/10.1007/978-981-19-9418-0_10

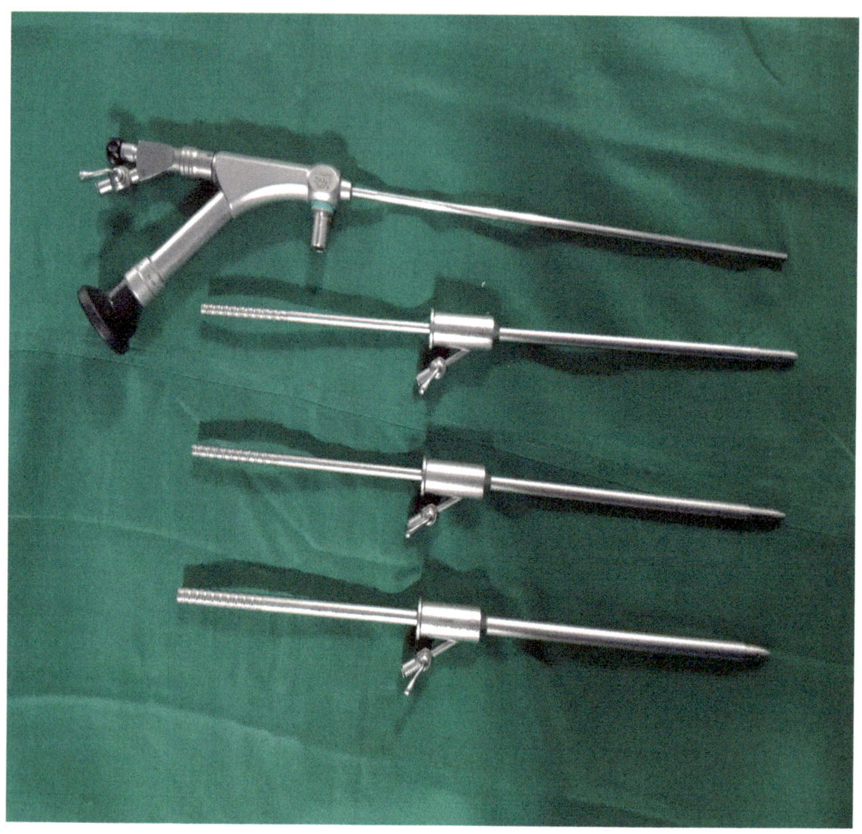

Fig. 10.1 Miniperc system—shows telescope of 12 F size and 3 sheaths with its dilators

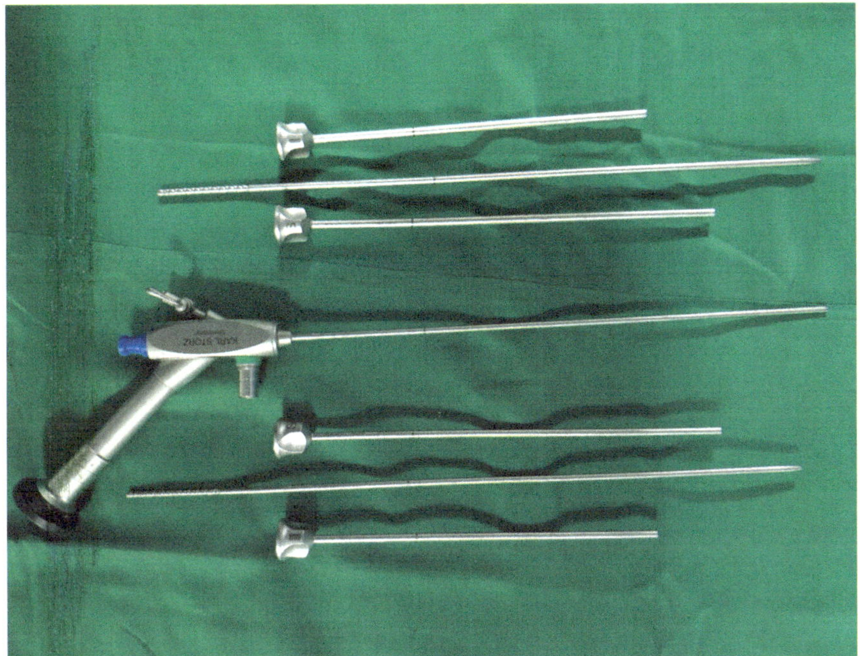

Fig. 10.2 Miniperc XS system—shows telescope of 7.5 F and sheath of 9.5 F with its dilator

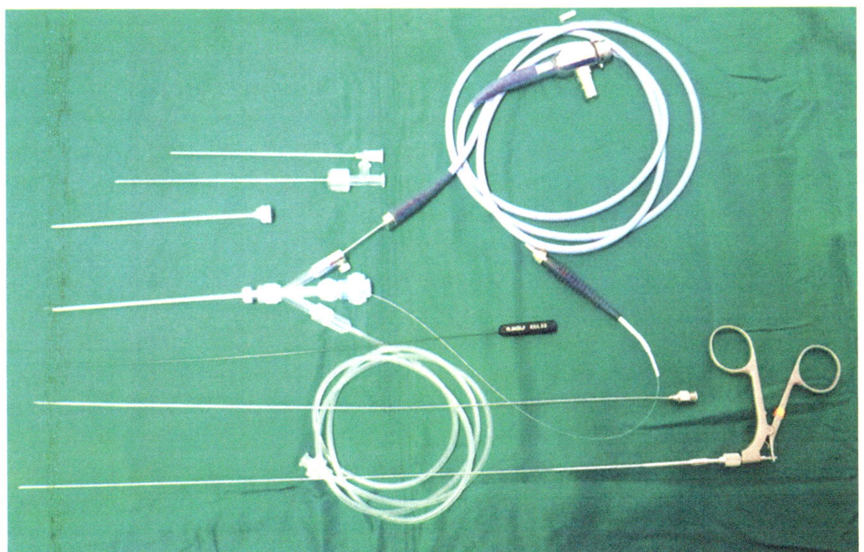

Fig. 10.3 Microperc system. Showing 16 G needle, telescope of 0.9 mm diameter

10.2 Indications [1, 2]

The standard indications are

1. Solitary stones usually less than 1.5 cm
2. Lower calyceal stones
3. Stones in the diverticula

As the use of this technology is spreading some of the operators have started using this technique for stones in urinary conduits, ectopic kidneys with stones, stones of larger size using 8 Fr sheaths and in children with urolithiasis and treatment for infundibular stenosis [3–7].

10.3 Microperc—The Technique

This system consists of single step percutaneous access to pelvicalyceal system. Once in the system, the stone dusting is achieved with holmium laser. The stone debris clears up with irrigation system (Fig. 10.3) [8, 9].

Though the preferred form of anesthesia is general anesthesia, some units have successfully performed this procedure with regional anesthesia. There are reports of use of Valdivia modified position [10] for this technique, The authors prefer to use the standard technique of supine introduction of ureteric catheter and then prone position for the puncture.

It is the practice of authors to use single step puncture using the "all seeing needle" while the assistant fills up the pelvicalyceal system with fluid filled with contrast. A similar method uses an ultrasound probe to use the standard puncture needle and a single step dilation to accommodate the 16 G needle. After the entry of Microperc, the stone is visualized. A 3-way adapter is then attached to the needle scope hub. The 3-way adapter allows the use of 200 or 272 micron fiber and the 0.9 mm flexible scope and the irrigation (Fig. 10.4). The preferred energy settings are 0.8 J and 8 Hz with effective Wattage being 6.4 W.

Some operators modified this instrumentation to use an outer sheath of 8 and 10 Fr. This allows more stability for extra mobility to do intrarenal manipulation. This new technique is called Mini Microperc and allows the use of 1.6 mm ultrasonic lithotripter and 3 Fr forceps to extract stones [3, 6]. In a study done in pediatric population, a further modification led to the use of 14 G (6.6 Fr) Angiocath as an Amplatz sheath [11].

Miniaturization of instruments, puncture needles, sheaths, and energy sources have led to decreased complication rates and morbidity associated with the procedure [12]. The technique of Microperc does not require any different facet of learning since the calyceal access techniques remain the same, i.e., fluoroscopy or the ultrasound guidance.

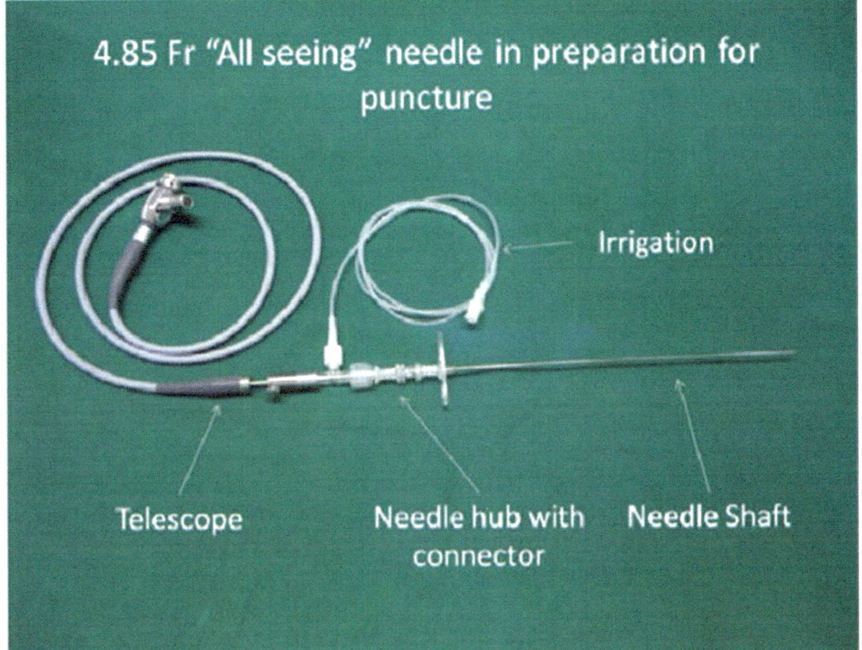

Fig. 10.4 The all-seeing needle

10.3.1 Clearance

Desai et al. used the all-seeing needle introduced by Bader et al. [8, 9, 13]. The 10 patients in their study had the mean stone size of 14.3 mm. The authors reported 89% success rate. Besides this the largest of the studies are the ones by Ganpule et al. [14] and by Hatipoglu et al. [15]. The technique reports high success rate ranging from 82% in larger series to 100% in the smaller ones.

10.3.2 Hospital Stays

As the exit strategy of tubeless approach leads to shorter hospital stay, the average stays in reported series are 1–2 days only [16].

10.3.3 Complications Associated with Microperc

The reported complications of this techniques are

1. Bleeding related to puncture and dilation
2. Exposure to radiation

3. Clavien–Dindo grades of lower grade accounting for fever, renal colic and UTI
4. Urinary extravasation and the need for JJ stent placement
5. Steinstrasse needing JJ placement

Hatipoglu et al. [15] in their series have even routinely stented patients with >2 cm in the preoperative period. It seems plausible that energy settings performing "dusting," that is high frequency and low energy might bring down the incidence of these complications related to larger stone debris and obstruction of the upper urinary tract.

The technical difficulties encountered are poor visibility in case of bleeding. Stone migration in the larger dilated pelvicalyceal system also adds to the difficulties in these cases. The remedies for this problem are conversion to Miniperc. This not only allows larger size of access sheath to be used but also allows use of larger ultrasonic lithotripter to bring about affective lithotripsy and renal of clots as well [9, 12, 17, 18]. The operative time is shortened significantly as well.

10.4 How Does this Technique Fare When Compared to Other Methods?

When compared with ESWL in pediatric population, Hatipoglu et al. found lower retreatment rates for Microperc [19]. They reported lower ancillary procedures and high success rates.

In comparison to RIRS, Sabnis et al. found similar clearance rates and complication rates very similar in both groups [20]. In similar studies by Armagan and Fata, the success rates of Microperc was significantly more with better safety profile [21, 22]. These studies had stone sizes less than 2 cm.

Karatag et al. [23] reported a study in pediatric population of Microperc ($n = 56$) and Miniperc ($n = 63$) with stone size ranging between 10 and 20 mm. The stone-free rates in both the groups (92.8% vs 93.6%, $P = 0.0673$) were similar at first-month follow-up. The difference in mean hemoglobin drop and hospital stay was in favor of Microperc. Stays in hours were 43.0 ± 15.4 vs 68.5 ± 31.7 h ($P < 0.001$). The overall complication rates ($P = 0.159$) were the same in both groups. The 3 complications (5.3%) observed in the Microperc group were saline extravasation ($n = 1$) requiring percutaneous abdominal drainage (Clavien grade IIIb) and persistent renal colic ($n = 2$) requiring stent insertion in the Microperc group (Clavien grade IIIb). The complication rate reported in the Miniperc group was 12.6%, with hemorrhage requiring blood transfusion in 5 patients and one patient each requiring ureterorenoscopy and double J stenting (Clavien grade IIIb study), medical therapy for pyrexia (Clavien grade I), and antibiotic for urinary tract infection postoperatively (Clavien grade II). The authors concluded that Microperc may be preferred as an alternative to Miniperc for the treatment of pediatric kidney stones of sizes 10–20 mm with comparable success and complication rates, as well as shorter hospitalization and fluoroscopy times. The drawback of this series is however the fact that it was a retrospective series.

Tok et al. [24] reported a comparative study between Mini and Microperc. Their conclusion was similar stone-free rates 86.2% vs 82.5%. The mean Hb drop however was in favor of Micro Perc group (1.96% vs 3.98% p value less than 0.001). The duration of hospitalization also was significantly less in microperc group (1.55 days vs 2.63 days, p value less than 0.01).

10.5 Conclusions

This new technique adheres to all basic points of a conventional PCNL, i.e., a perfect puncture and small dilation of tract which minimizes the complications and morbidity. We are seeing reports of larger stone volumes and better clearances with the novel tubeless approach [25]. As energy sources undergo developments such as refined and finer laser fibers we shall see a surge in the use of this modality.

This innovation in percutaneous stone management appears to be another milestone in the quest for **"knife to cannula to needle to nothing"** [26].

Acknowledgements Nil.

Disclosures Nil.

References

1. Preminger GM. Micro-percutaneous nephrolithotomy (micro-PNL) vs retrograde intra-renal surgery (RIRS): dealer's choice? The devil is in the details. BJU Int. 2013;112(3):280–1.
2. Ganpule AP, Bhattu AS, Desai M. PCNL in the twenty-first century: role of microperc, Miniperc, and Ultraminiperc. World J Urol. 2015;33(2):235–40.
3. Sabnis RB, Ganesamoni R, Ganpule AP, Mishra S, Vyas J, Jagtap J, et al. Current role of microperc in the management of small renal calculi. Indian J Urol. 2013;29:214–8.
4. Armagan A, Tepeler A, Silay MS, et al. Micropercutaneous nephrolithotomy in the treatment of moderate-size renal calculi. J Endourol. 2013;27:177–81.
5. Ganesamoni R, Sabnis RB, Mishra S, Desai MR. Microperc for the management of renal calculi in pelvic ectopic kidneys. Indian J Urol. 2013;29:257–9.
6. Sabnis RB, Chhabra JS, Ganpule AP, Abrol S, Desai MR. Current role of PCNL in pediatric urolithiasis. Curr Urol Rep. 2014;15(7):1–8.
7. Sancaktutar AA, Adanur S, Ziypak T, Hatipoglu NK, Bodakcı MN, Soylemez H, Ozbey I. Micropercutaneous nephrolithotomy in the management of bilateral renal stones in a 7-month-old infant: the youngest case in the literature. Urol Int. 2014;96(2):238–40.
8. Bader MJ, Gratzke C, Seitz M, Sharma R, Stief CG, Desai M. The "all-seeing needle": initial results of an optical puncture system confirming access in percutaneous nephrolithotomy. Eur Urol. 2011;59:1054–9.
9. Desai MR, Sharma R, Mishra S, et al. Single-step percutaneous nephrolithotomy (microperc): the initial clinical report. J Urol. 2011;186:140–5.
10. Karatag T, Tepeler A, Buldu I, Akcay M, Tosun M, Istanbulluoglu MO, Armagan A. Is micro-percutaneous nephrolithotomy surgery technically feasible and efficient under spinal anesthesia? Urolithiasis. 2015;43:249–54.
11. Penbegul N, Bodakci MN, Hatipoglu NK, Sancaktutar AA, Atar M, Cakmakci S, et al. Micro sheath for microperc: 14 gauge angiocath. J Endourol. 2013;27:835–9.

12. Kukreja R, Desai M, Patel S, et al. Factors affecting blood loss during percutaneous nephrolithotomy: prospective study. J Endourol. 2004;18:715–22.
13. Bader M, Gratzke C, Schlenker B, et al. 1890 The "all-seeing needle"—an optical puncture system confirming percutaneous access in PNL. J Urol. 2010;183:e734.
14. Ganpule A, Chhabra JS, Kore V, Mishra S, Sabnis R, Desai M. Factors predicting outcomes of micropercutaneous nephrolithotomy: results from a large single-centre experience. BJU Int. 2016;117(3):478–83. https://doi.org/10.1111/bju.13263.
15. Hatipoglu NK, Tepeler A, Buldu I, Atis G, Bodakci MN, Sancaktutar AA, Silay MS, et al. Initial experience of micro-percutaneous nephrolithotomy in the treatment of renal calculi in 140 renal units. Urolithiasis. 2014;42(2):159–64.
16. Akman T, Binbay M, Yuruk E, Sari E, Seyrek M, Kaba M, Berberoglu Y, Muslumanoglu AY. Tubeless procedure is most important factor in reducing length of hospitalization after percutaneous nephrolithotomy: results of univariable and multivariable models. Urology. 2011;77(2):299–304. https://doi.org/10.1016/j.urology.2010.06.060.
17. Tepeler A, Armagan A, Sancaktutar AA, et al. The role of microperc in the treatment of symptomatic lower pole renal calculi. J Endourol. 2013;27:13–8.
18. Piskin MM, Guven S, Kilinc M, Arslan M, Goger E, Ozturk A. Preliminary, favorable experience with microperc in kidney and bladder stones. J Endourol. 2012;26(11):1443–7.
19. Hatipoglu NK, Sancaktutar AA, Tepeler A, et al. Comparison of shockwave lithotripsy and microperc for treatment of kidney stones in children. J Endourol. 2013;27(9):1141–6.
20. Sabnis RB, Ganesamoni R, Doshi A, Ganpule AP, Jagtap J, Desai MR. Micropercutaneous nephrolithotomy (microperc) vs retrograde intrarenal surgery for the management of small renal calculi: a randomized controlled trial. BJU Int. 2013;112:355–61.
21. Ramón de Fata F, García-Tello A, Andrés G, Redondo C, Meilán E, Gimbernat H, Angulo JC. Comparative study of retrograde intrarenal surgery and micropercutaneous nephrolithotomy in the treatment of intermediate-sized kidney stones. Actas Urol Esp. 2014;38(9):576–83. https://doi.org/10.1016/j.acuro.2014.04.004.
22. Armagan A, Karatag T, Buldu I, Tosun M, Basibuyuk I, Istanbulluoglu MO, Tepeler A. Comparison of flexible ureterorenoscopy and micropercutaneous nephrolithotomy in the treatment for moderately size lower-pole stones. World J Urol. 2015;33:1827–31.
23. Karatag T, Buldu I, Inan R, Istanbulluoglu MO. Is micropercutaneous nephrolithotomy technique really efficacious for the treatment of moderate size renal calculi? Yes. Urol Int. 2015;95(1):9–14.
24. Tok A, Akbulut F, Buldu I, Karatag T, Kucuktopcu O, Gurbuz G, Istanbulluoglu O, Armagan A, Tepeler A, Tasci AI. Comparison of microperc and mini-percutaneous nephrolithotomy for medium-sized lower calyx stones. Urolithiasis. 2015;21:155–9.
25. Desai M. Editorial comment. J Urol. 2016;195(3):746. https://doi.org/10.1016/j.juro.2015.07.125.
26. Clayman RV. From knife to needle to nothing: the waning of the wound. Braz J Urol. 2001;27:209–14.

11 Supine PCNL

Ravindra Sabnis and Abhishek Singh

Percutaneous nephrolithotomy (PCNL) has been practiced since four decades now. During in this time, this procedure has undergone significant evolution. All the effort has been directed to improve stone clearance with least possible morbidity. As individual surgeon's expertise went on improving so did the complexity of cases. In an endeavor to decrease morbidity and improve stone clearance, PCNL was tried in different positions. Godwin et al. had described the first percutaneous access to kidney in prone position and Fernstorm et al. described their first PCNL in prone position [1, 2]. PCNL in prone position pretty much became the standard of care as it provided a wide surgical field, good space for movement of nephroscope, upper pole access was possible with a low risk of injury to pleura, lung, and adjacent organs.

Prone position is a matter of concern for the anesthesia team as the airway is difficult to manage, adverse hemodynamic changes could occur, with a risk of associated iatrogenic injuries, pressure injuries, ophthalmic injuries. Also, prone position is either very difficult to achieve or not possible in morbidly obese patients and patients with musculoskeletal deformities. These potential problems of prone position gave rise to PCNL in other positions.

Various positions for PCNL have been described. Grasso et al. described PCNL in lateral decubitus, but it was Valdivia Uria who first described PCNL in supine position [3]. This Spanish group popularized supine PCNL over a decade by producing consistent data over this period. Finally, the world started accepting this supine PCNL. Though PCNL is still done by majority of urologist in prone position. The debate on patient positioning is endless, is it that we all are used to doing prone PCNL from its inception and therefore are reluctant to see the advantages of supine PCNL.

The question whether supine PCNL is as good as prone PCNL would be answered in this current chapter.

R. Sabnis (✉) · A. Singh
Department of Urology, MPUH, Nadiad, India

S. R. Shivde (ed.), *Techniques in Percutaneous Renal Stone Surgery*, https://doi.org/10.1007/978-981-19-9418-0_11

11.1 Supine Patient Positioning

Supine PCNL is not truly supine as it has many variations described by various authors, we shall try to describe a few of them

1. Supine PCNL can be done in pure supine position, without any sandbag or bolster under the lumbar region. If this position is to be used, patient should be positioned at the lateral edge of the table and the table should not have any metal bars by the side [4, 5].
2. Valdivia position (Fig. 11.1): Prerequisite: a radiolucent operation table and a 3-L water bag. Patient is placed either in pure supine position or split leg position, with both legs flexed. A 3-L water bag is placed under the concerned lumbar region. Ipsilateral arm is flexed and supported on the thorax. Patients flank should be at the edge of the surgical table [3, 6].
3. Galdakao-modified supine Valdivia position (GMSV) (Fig. 11.2): Described by Ibarluzea et al. from Spain. In this position. Patient is in dorsal decubitus with the limbs supported on stirrups—the ipsilateral limb is extended, and the contralateral limb is flexed [7].
4. Oblique position: Patient is maintained in oblique position by 2 gel pads one under the hip and the other under the shoulder. The proponents of this position believe that this gives a larger freedom of movement for the nephroscope [8].

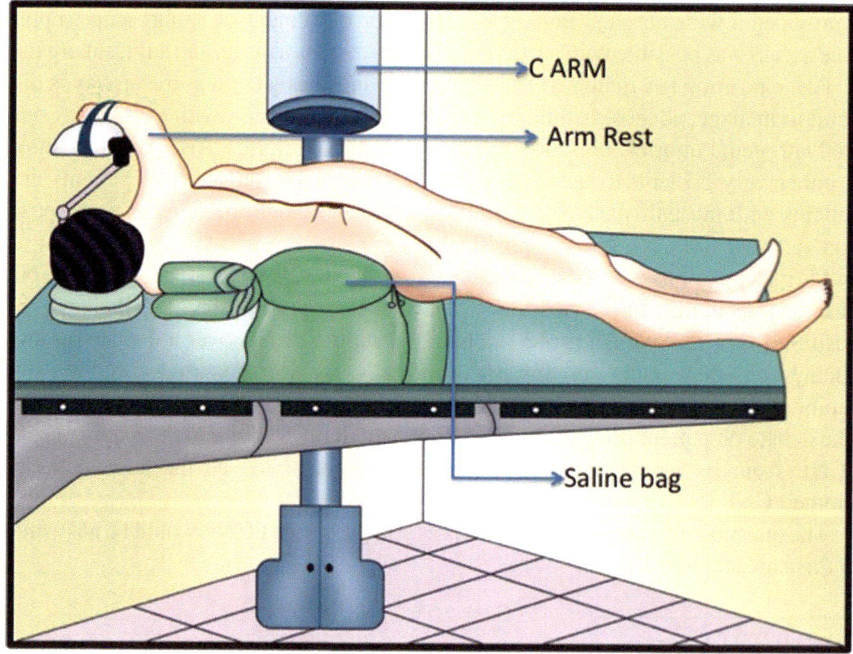

Fig. 11.1 Classical Valdivia position

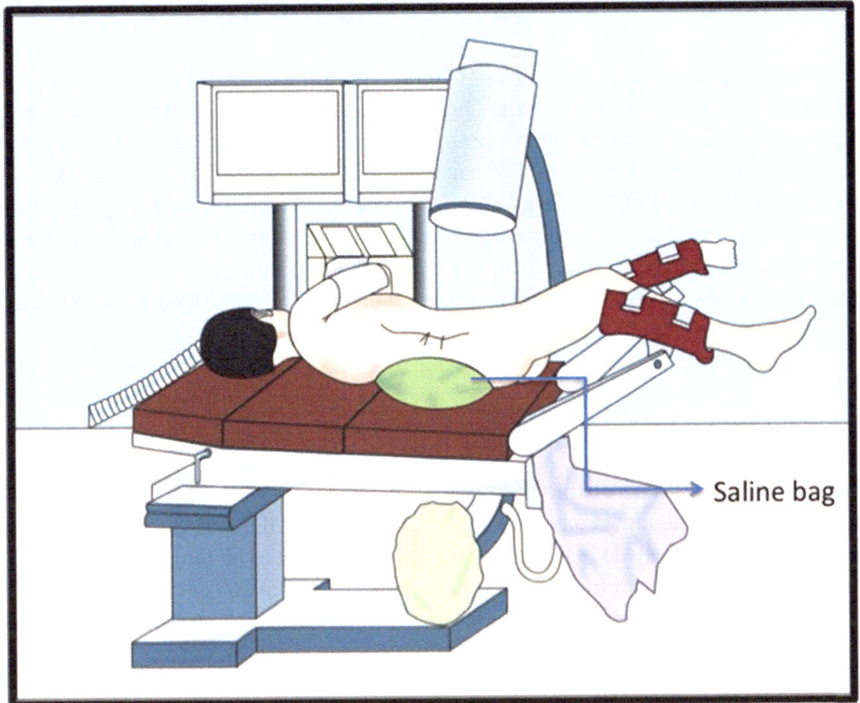

Fig. 11.2 Galdakao-modified supine Valdivia position

5. Finally, Perez-Castro et al. described position in which, patients are placed in lithotomy position with lumbar fossa supported as described above, only difference is that ipsilateral limb is elevated and contralateral descended [9].

11.2 Operating Room Set-Up for Supine PCNL

1. Operating table—should be radiolucent, should not have side metal bars, and should have facility for placing stirrups, which could be adjusted in height
2. Gel pads, 3-L saline bags, sandbags for placement under the lumbar fossa
3. A pair of stirrups
4. Gel pads, cotton roll for padding the pressure points
5. Two sets of endo-vision (optional) if simultaneous retrograde and antegrade procedure is planned

11.3 Patient Positioning and Marking (Figs. 11.1 and 11.2)

Posterior axillary line is marked in standing and sitting position, as it would get distorted in oblique position. After induction of anesthesia, patient is positioned supine, and the concerned side is brought to the edge of the table. We keep the patient on a sandbag below the lumbar fossa and both the limbs are supported on stirrups, ipsilateral limb is extended, lowered and contralateral limb is flexed, elevated as compared to opposite side. All the pressure points are padded. Ipsilateral limb is kept flexed and folded over the chest or head. Important anatomical landmarks, namely 12th rib, iliac crest is marked with a skin marker. The flank and genitalia are scrubbed and draped.

11.4 Operative Room Setup (Fig. 11.3)

All monitors should be visible to the surgeon when he is doing per urethral procedure as well as when he is working in the lumbar area. All the lines like light cable, suction and lithotripsy device cable or the laser fiber should be tangle free. If simultaneous antegrade and retrograde access is contemplated, two sets of monitors with light, camera and scopes should be available. The operating surgeon is in sitting position while doing the puncture.

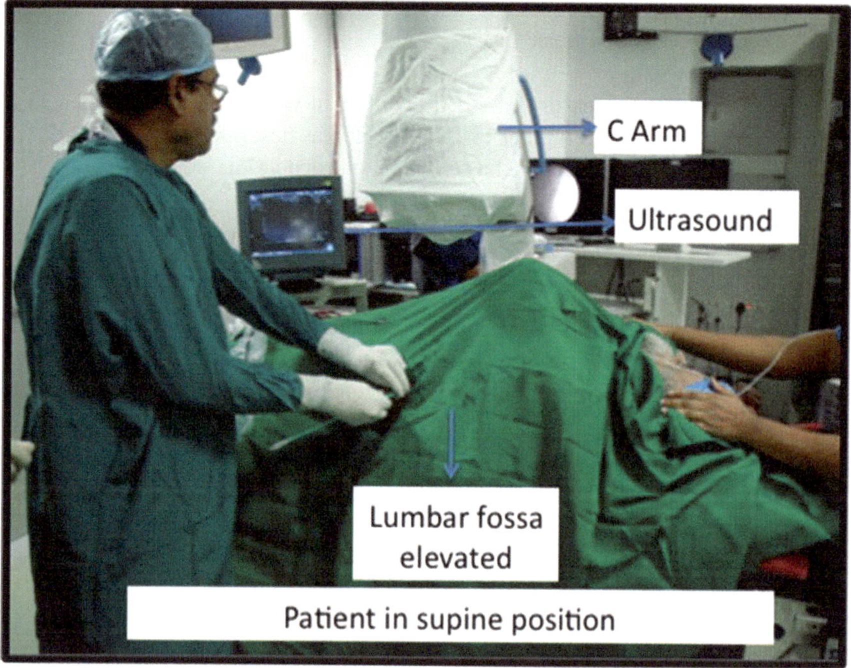

Fig. 11.3 Photograph of operative room setup and patient position for PCNL in supine position

11.5 Operative Procedure

The lumbar region is screened with ultrasound, using a 3.5 MHz probe and the direction of the needle is ascertained. Most of the ultrasound machines have a puncture attachment and guide, which can be used to visualize the puncture trajectory and finally can be used to puncture. Simultaneously C-arm is also positioned, and the kidney visualized after injecting the contrast. The lower calyx is last to fill, and this problem can be overcome by placing the patient in reverse Trendelenburg position, also the amount of contract injected should be little more and under pressure, but one must be careful not to cause any extravasations. Gentle palpation of the kidney causes even distribution of the contrast. In case of an obstructing calculus, any communicating calyx can be punctured and then antegrade dye injected to opacify the lower calyx.

The calyx to be punctured is selected and marked; a point on pre-marked posterior axillary line is elected which is in line with the selected calyx. Using any of the above imaging modalities surgeon begins to puncture. The direction of the needle is upward (Figs. 11.4 and 11.5a) as opposed to downwards in prone (Fig. 11.5b). Puncture is carried out using an 18 G needle. The needle is inserted in an ascending direction toward the desired calyx (Fig. 11.5a). After the skin and the muscular layers are pierced, the renal capsule is engaged and the kidney is jiggled. If the desired calyx moves and buckles or there is indentation of cup of the calyx (known as the fovea sign), the surgeon can be sure that his direction and depth are correct. When

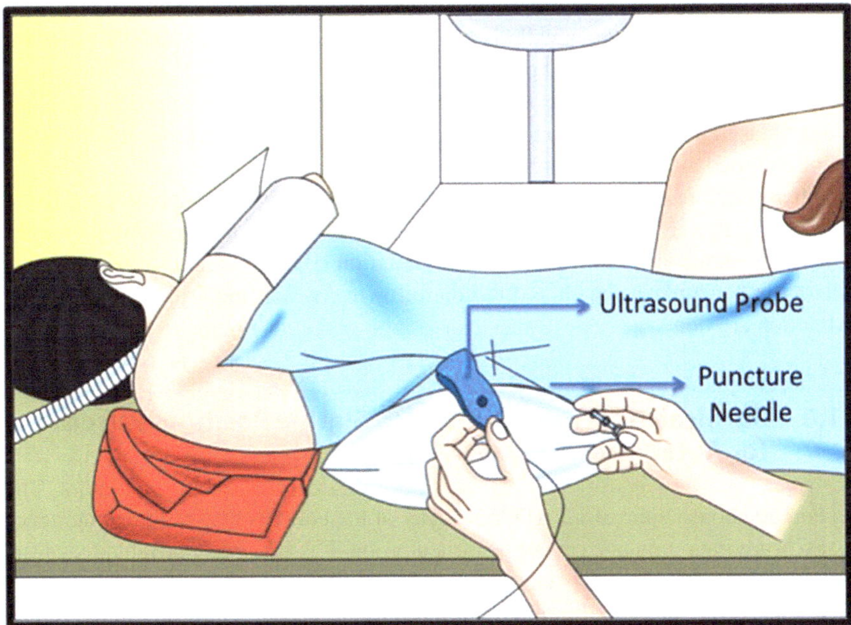

Fig. 11.4 Ultrasound guided puncture in supine position

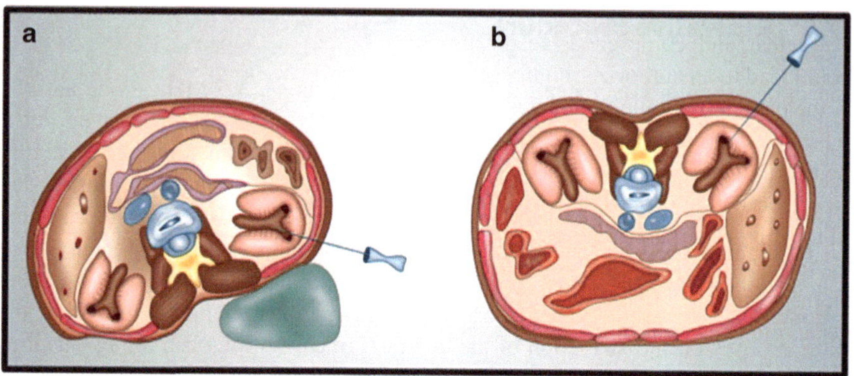

Fig. 11.5 (**a**) Orientation of needle while puncturing in supine position. (**b**) Showing orientation of needle while puncturing in prone position

the above does not happen, the surgeon should go superficial or deep with his needle and again look for the movement of calyx by trial and error. Once the calyx buckles, the needle is advanced till surgeon gets a giveaway feeling. The stylet of puncture needle is withdrawn, and efflux of clear urine conforms a correct puncture.

In case of an incorrect puncture, surgeon should move the needle up and down and observe the movement of the contrast filled calyx. If the needle is below/posterior to the calyx, the calyx will move anteriorly when the tip of the needle is moved up and if the needle is above/anterior to the calyx then, the calyx will move posteriorly when the tip of the needle is moved down. Common mistake in these punctures is that the direction of the needle is horizontal rather than ascending. Most of the punctures are anterior calyceal punctures in supine position. The X-rays are perpendicular to the needle and calyx; hence their movements are better appreciated. There is a decreased need for rotation of C-arm to 30° but one may still use it if puncture is not obtained after 3–4 attempts.

After puncture contrast is injected to confirm the entry of the needle through the cup of the calyx. Following this a guide wire is passed, the tract is dilated over the guide wire using desired method of tract dilatation (Balloon, telescopic or Amplatz dilator) and Amplatz sheath is placed, following which nephroscopy and stone extraction are done.

11.6 Surgical Indications for Which Supine Position is Used for Antegrade Access to Kidney

1. Percutaneous nephrostomy (PCN): Many of the patients who require emergency PCN are in uremia and cannot be turned prone. It is extremely advantageous and lifesaving to do these procedures in supine position.
2. Percutaneous nephrolithotomy (PCNL): Percutaneous nephrolithotomy can be done with ease and many advantages using this position.

3. Endoscopic Combined Intrarenal Surgery (ECIRS) [10]. In these types of procedures, two surgeons simultaneously access the pelvicalyceal system (PCS) via antegrade and retrograde route. One surgeon punctures the PCS antegradely and introduces a rigid nephroscope to visualize the PCS and the second surgeon does a flexible ureterorenoscopy and accesses the PCS. GMSV position works well for this approach.

   Potential uses and advantages of ECIRS

   (a) Patients with upper ureteric calculus with renal calculus can be managed with this technique.
   (b) Surgeon doing the ureterorenoscopy can collect the stone from different location and pass it to the surgeon doing the rigid nephroscopy (popularly known as **Passing the ball**) thereby reducing the number of percutaneous tracts.
   (c) Stones, which are lodged in the calyces, which are parallel to the punctured calyx, can be extracted using this technique.
   (d) Migration of the fragmented stones to the upper ureter can be prevented by presence of scope as well as the irrigation from ureteroscope.
   (e) Irrigation from the ureteroscope can help in improving the vision.
   (f) A comprehensive check nephroscopy can be performed using flexible ureteroscope at the end of the surgery.
   (g) At the end of the procedure ureter can be visualized for clots, edema, and stone fragments, this might help the surgeon decide objective whether a double J (DJ) stent placement is required.
4. Transcutaneous retrograde puncture of PCS. This method was described by Hunter and Lawson [11, 12]. In this method, a ureterorenoscopy is done and the desired calyx is visualized, and a sharp flexible wire is passed through the calyx onto the skin. The wire is loaded with a small 6 Fr facial dilator antegradely and withdrawn. Now the sharp wire is withdrawn, and a soft floppy tip wire is parked into the PCS and tract is serially dilated.
5. Percutaneous endopyelotomy: Percutaneous endopyelotomy has been demonstrated in supine position. In a series of 280 patients, endopylelotomy was done in supine position in 19 patients [6]. Similarly, endoureterotomy can also be done in supine position antegradely.
6. Percutaneous tumor resection: Valdivia et al. have described 2 cases of antegrade tumor resection in supine position in their series of 280 patients. This may be of importance as these patients may require simultaneous diagnostic cystoscopy, flexible ureteroscopy, and antegrade access for diagnosis and treatment of upper tract transitional cell carcinoma.
7. Supine position antegrade access has the potential to be combined with laparoscopy in situations like pyeloplasty, ureteric re-implantation, and stone surgery for ectopically placed kidneys.

11.7 Advantages of Doing PCNL in Supine Position

1. **Advantages to the urologist**
   (a) Surgeon operates in a sitting position, which is more comfortable and ergonomically better.
   (b) There is a decreased radiation exposure to the finger of the operating surgeon.
   (c) Movement of calyx is better visualized, as the X-rays are perpendicular to the calyx.
   (d) Proponents believe that puncturing in supine position is easier.
   (e) In obese patients in the above-described position, the pannus of fat gets displaced to the opposite side decreasing stone to skin distance.
   (f) Simultaneous antegrade and retrograde access is possible.
   (g) The direction of the Amplatz sheath is downwards; this helps drainage by gravity and creates a low-pressure system. This also facilitates stone extraction by gravity and by Whirlpool effect or Bernoulli's effect.
   (h) Supine position gives more space for movement of endourological equipment.
   (i) Total surgical time is decreased in supine position. The increased in time in prone position is attributed to change in position of the patient at the beginning and end of the procedure [13].
2. **Decreased anesthetic and positioning risk** [14]
   (a) Airway management is easier in supine position, and there is no risk of accidental removal of endotracheal tube while changing the position of patient.
   (b) Supine position is better tolerated in regional anesthesia.
   (c) Supine position is more physiological as there is no compression of inferior vena cava as diaphragm is not pulled up. Hence the incidence of cardiorespiratory embarrassment decreases.
   (d) As the patient is more comfortable in this position it is possible to do PCNL in regional or local anesthesia with sedation.
   (e) Iatrogenic risk of displacing the intravenous lines, electrodes, and urethral catheters is eliminated.
   (f) Iatrogenic injuries associated with prone positioning, neuropraxia, joint dislocation, pressure sores, and corneal ulcers can be avoided.
3. **Logistic advantages**

   Surgeon and assistants have to scrub only once; same set of drape is used for urethral catheterization and PCNL. There is no hassle of placing and removing the stirrups, neither is an extension table for placing patients' legs is required. Manpower required to turn the patient prone also decreases in supine position. The equipment has to be plugged and unplugged, moved round about, causing wear and tear in prone position which does not happen in supine position.

   All the above may significantly decrease the cost of the procedure.
4. **Decrease in complication rate**
   (a) Colonic injuries: As the colon gets displaced posteriorly in prone position, there is an increased incidence of colonic perforation in prone position. This

has been proven in computed tomography studies. There is a definite decrease in the risk of colonic injuries in supine position [6]. In a series of 287 patients with antegrade access in supine position, there was no colonic injury. In a review article comparing 9 series of PCNL in supine position, there was no report of colonic injury [15].

(b) Incidence of bleeding: Transfusion rates vary from 1.5 to 9% in various series of supine PCNL [16–18] and rate of angioembolization is up to 0.5% in various series [15]. Theoretically the risk of bleeding decreases as the punctures pass through the cup of the calyx more often than not. As there in no vena cava compression, there is decreased congestion and bleeding [15].

11.8 Success Rates of PCNL in Supine Position

The stone-free rates in PCNL in prone and supine position were compared in a randomized controlled trail by De Sio et al. They reported a stone-free rate of 88.7% in supine position as compared to 91.6% in prone position [13]. Shoma et al. in their study had a similar stone clearance rate for both the positions [18].

11.8.1 Is Supine Position Effective in Special Situations?

1. **Upper calyceal puncture:** Approaching the superior calyx, which is medially placed, is difficult in supine position. On the left side approaching superior calyx becomes more difficult [17, 19]. In cases with the patients having wide hips and narrow calyces, it is not possible to enter the superior calyx with rigid nephroscope, a flexible nephroscope should be used. Also, superior calyx can be approached in a retrograde manner and stone clearance assisted. Some authors do not find it difficult to gain an upper pole access in supine position.
2. **Managing upper ureteric calculus:** Ideal puncture to access upper ureter is superior calyx. We face the problems associated with superior calyceal puncture in managing upper ureteric stones. But simultaneous retrograde access can be used to push the stone into PCS using varied types of ureteric catheters and injection of saline. Rigid ureteroscopes can be used to fragment the stones simultaneously and push the stones in PCS. Flexible ureteroscope can be a handful if available in these situations.
3. **Staghorn calculus** [20]: Wang et al. demonstrated that PCNL in supine position is feasible in staghorn calculus. In their series, the stone clearance rate was 83.3%, with a mean hemoglobin drop of 2.12 g. No blood transfusions were required, and there was no adjacent organ injury in the above series.
4. **Multiple punctures:** In patients requiring multiple puncture, supine position is difficult as the working area decreases and superior calyceal punctures become difficult.

11.8.2 Disadvantages of Supine Position

1. Approaching the superior calyx, which is medially placed, is difficult in supine position as described above.
2. The kidneys are mobile in supine position therefore there may be difficulty in puncturing and dilatation. But since these kidneys become more mobile, we can perform an infracostal superior calyceal puncture more easily. The movement of the kidney can be restricted by contralateral abdominal compression.
3. Due to gravity, the PCS is always in a collapsed state making nephroscopy slightly difficult. This can overcome by placing a stopper or gauze tied around the nephroscope.
4. Lower pole calyx takes longer time to fill with contrast, but this can be overcome with simple measures described earlier in text.

11.9 Conclusion

Supine positions for PCNL are more physiological and have a better safety profile from anesthetic standpoint. It is a highly effective procedure in high risk and morbidly obese patients. It is safe, replicable, reduces total operative time, and gives surgeon an opportunity for simultaneous antegrade and retrograde access. It is for sure that PCNL in supine position has advantages, but it will not be able to totally replace PCNL in prone position in situations where upper calyceal and multiple punctures are required for stone clearance.

Acknowledgements Nil.

Disclosure Nil.

References

1. Goodwin WE, Casey WC, Woolf W. Percutaneous trocar (needle) nephrostomy in hydronephrosis. J Am Med Assoc. 1955;157(11):891–4.
2. Fernström I, Johansson B. Percutaneous pyelolithotomy. A new extraction technique. Scand J Urol Nephrol. 1976;10(3):257.
3. Uria JV, Santamaria EL, Rodriguez SV, Llop JT, Baquero GA, Lassa JA. Percutaneous nephrolithotomy: simplified technique (preliminary report). Arch Esp Urol. 1987;40:177–80.
4. Melchert E, Junior JD. New technique to perform percutaneous nephrolithotripsy total dorsal decubitus. Actas Urol Esp. 2010;34(8):726–9.
5. Falahatkar S, Allahkhah A. Recent developments in percutaneous nephrolithotomy: benefits of the complete supine position. UroToday Int J. 2010;3(2):3.
6. Valdivia JG, Valer J, Villarroya S, López JA, Bayo A, Lanchares E, Rubio E. Why is percutaneous nephroscopy still performed with the patient prone? J Endourol. 1990;4(3):269–77.
7. Ibarluzea G, Scoffone CM, Cracco CM, Poggio M, Porpiglia F, Terrone C, Astobieta A, Camargo I, Gamarra M, Tempia A, Valdivia Uria JG. Supine Valdivia and modified lithot-

omy position for simultaneous anterograde and retrograde endourological access. BJU Int. 2007;100(1):233–6.

8. Cormio L, Annese P, Corvasce T, De Siati M, Turri FP, Lorusso F, Pentimone S, Perrone A, Carrieri G. Percutaneous nephrostomy in supine position. Urology. 2007;69(2):377–80.
9. Perez Castro E, Martinez Pineiro JA, La ureterorrenoscopia transuretral. Un actual proceder urológico. Arch Esp Urol. 1980;33:445–60.
10. Scoffone CM, Cracco CM, Cossu M, Grande S, Poggio M, Scarpa RM. Endoscopic combined intrarenal surgery in Galdakao-modified supine Valdivia position: a new standard for percutaneous nephrolithotomy? Eur Urol. 2008;54(6):1393–403.
11. Lawson RK, Murphy JB, Taylor AJ, Jacobs SC. Retrograde method for percutaneous access to kidney. Urology. 1983;22(6):580–2.
12. Hunter PT, Hawkins IF, Finlayson B, Nanni G, Senior D. Hawkins–Hunter retrograde transcutaneous nephrostomy: a new technique. Urology. 1983;22(6):583–7.
13. De Sio M, Autorino R, Quarto G, Calabrò F, Damiano R, Giugliano F, Mordente S, D'Armiento M. Modified supine versus prone position in percutaneous nephrolithotomy for renal stones treatable with a single percutaneous access: a prospective randomized trial. Eur Urol. 2008;54(1):196–203.
14. Manohar T, Jain P, Desai M. Supine percutaneous nephrolithotomy: effective approach to high-risk and morbidly obese patients. J Endourol. 2007;21(1):44–9.
15. Basiri A, Mohammadi SM. Supine percutaneous nephrolithotomy, is it really effective? A systematic review of literature. Urol J. 2009;6(2):73–7.
16. Uria JV, Gerhold JV, López JL, Rodriguez SV, Navarro CA, Fabián MR, Bazalo JR, Elipe MS. Technique and complications of percutaneous nephroscopy: experience with 557 patients in the supine position. J Urol. 1998;160(6):1975–8.
17. Ng MT, Sun WH, Cheng CW, Chan ES. Supine position is safe and effective for percutaneous nephrolithotomy. J Endourol. 2004;18(5):469–74.
18. Shoma AM, Eraky I, El-Kenawy MR, El-Kappany HA. Percutaneous nephrolithotomy in the supine position: technical aspects and functional outcome compared with the prone technique. Urology. 2002;60(3):388–92.
19. Rana AM, Bhojwani JP, Junejo NN, Bhagia SD. Tubeless PCNL with patient in supine position: procedure for all seasons? With comprehensive technique. Urology. 2008;71(4):581–5.
20. Wang Y, Hou Y, Jiang F, Wang Y, Wang C. Percutaneous nephrolithotomy for staghorn stones in patients with solitary kidney in prone position or in completely supine position: a single-center experience. Int Braz J Urol. 2012;38(6):788–94.

PCNL Complications

Complications in Percutaneous Renal Surgery

Abhay Rane and S. Segaran

12.1 Introduction, Incidence, and Classification

PCNL is a generally safe and effective procedure for the treatment of renal stones and has largely superseded open surgery as the recommended first-line treatment for large renal stones (>2 cm) [1, 2]. There has previously been considerable variation in the reported rate of complications, with overall rates ranging from as low as 3.7% to as high as 50–81% [3, 4]. However, it is accepted that most of these complications are clinically insignificant [4].

Accurate recording and classification of complications are essential for the purposes of audit and comparison. In the past, arbitrary classification of complications (such as "major" and "minor") could lead to confusion and discrepancies in reporting, with reported rates of complications varying widely between published series. Currently, standardized reporting of complications using the Clavien–Dindo system (Table 12.1) [6] is recommended. To minimize discrepancy in reporting complication grades, procedure-specific guidance on assigning complications in PCNL to complication grades is available (Table 12.2). Recent meta-analysis of data utilizing this system has provided an insight into contemporary complication rates in PCNL [5].

A. Rane (✉)
East Surrey Hospital, Redhill, UK
e-mail: a.rane1@nhs.net

S. Segaran
Damansara Specialist Hospital 2, Kuala Lumpur, Malaysia

S. R. Shivde (ed.), *Techniques in Percutaneous Renal Stone Surgery*,
https://doi.org/10.1007/978-981-19-9418-0_12

Table 12.1 Clavien–Dindo classification

		Incidence in PCNL [5]
Grade 1	Any deviation from the normal postoperative course without the need for pharmacologic treatment or surgical, endoscopic, and radiologic interventions. Allowed therapeutic regimens are drugs as antiemetics, antipyretics, analgesics, diuretics, electrolytes, and physiotherapy. This grade also includes wound infections opened at the bedside	11.4%
Grade 2	Complications requiring pharmacologic treatment with drugs other than such allowed for grade 1 complications. Blood transfusions and total parenteral nutrition are also included	7.1%
Grade 3	Complications requiring surgical, endoscopic, or radiologic intervention	
Grade 3a	Intervention not under general anaesthesia	2.7%
Grade 3b	Intervention under general anaesthesia	1.4%
Grade 4	Life-threatening complications (including central nervous system complications) requiring intensive care unit stay	
Grade 4a	Single organ dysfunction (including dialysis)	0.4%
Grade 4b	Multiorgan dysfunction	0.2%
Grade 5	Death of the patient	0.04%

Table 12.2 Categorization of percutaneous nephrolithotomy-specific complications according to Clavien–Dindo classification score [4]

Clavien–Dindo score	Complication-management definitions
None	Normal postoperative trajectory without any unexpected deviation Blocked nephrostomy managed by removal of nephrostomy (without consequences) Nephrostomy tube discomfort that requires removal of nephrostomy Postoperative pain managed by nonopioid analgesics
1	Postoperative pain managed by opioid with or without adjunct analgesic regimen Postoperative fever (>38.0 °C) managed by observation without antibiotics Deranged renal function that requires IV fluid management only Bleeding managed using IV fluid without need for blood transfusion Bleeding that requires a single episode of nephrostomy clamping Bleeding that requires skin compression/pressure dressing Renal pelvic perforation managed by watchful waiting Urine leakage managed by watchful waiting Ureteric clot managed by watchful waiting Bladder retention without blood clot that requires bladder catheterization Pneumothorax managed by watchful waiting Hydrothorax managed by watchful waiting Displaced nephrostomy managed by watchful waiting Intestinal obstruction managed without nasogastric decompression

Table 12.2 (continued)

Clavien–Dindo score	Complication-management definitions
2	Bleeding requiring blood transfusion Nephrostomy site cellulitis managed by antibiotics Symptomatic UTI managed using antibiotics Postoperative fever (>38.0 °C) managed with antibiotics in the ward Colon perforation managed conservatively using IV fluid and antibiotics without controlled colocutaneous fistula Postoperative ileus managed by nasogastric decompression Postoperative pneumonia managed by antibiotics Heart failure (NYHA I and II) requiring management by medications in the ward Hyposaturation managed by oxygen in the ward Pulmonary oedema managed by diuretics Supraventricular arrhythmias requiring antiarrhythmic medications Minor atelectasis requiring medical management
3a	Febrile UTI or suspected sepsis without organ failure requiring supportive therapy and enhanced monitoring Bleeding requiring multiple bladder washouts/irrigations Bleeding managed with haemostatic agents placed endoscopically Bleeding that requires multiple episodes of nephrostomy clamping (>4 h apart) Bleeding managed by postoperative ureteric stenting without general anaesthesia Bleeding managed by postoperative placement of new larger-bore nephrostomy tamponade Colon perforation managed conservatively using controlled colocutaneous fistula Hemothorax managed by intercostal draining under local anaesthesia Hydrothorax managed by intercostal draining under local anaesthesia Pneumothorax managed by intercostal draining under local anaesthesia Renal pelvic perforation managed by prolonged nephrostomy tube or postoperative placement of nephrostomy Renal pelvic perforation managed by ureteric stenting without general anaesthesia Ureteric clot obstruction managed by ureteric stenting without general anaesthesia Urine leakage managed by postoperative placement of a new nephrostomy tube Urine leakage managed by ureteric stenting without general anaesthesia Blocked nephrostomy managed by ureteric stenting without general anaesthesia Misplaced double-J stent managed by repositioning Displaced nephrostomy requiring ureteric stenting without general anaesthesia Perirenal abscess managed by percutaneous drainage

(continued)

Table 12.2 (continued)

Clavien–Dindo score	Complication-management definitions
3b	Bleeding managed by angioembolisation Bleeding managed by nephrectomy Colon perforation managed by colostomy Ureteric stricture managed by balloon dilation Avulsion of the ureteropelvic junction managed by surgical repair Retained nephrostomy requiring removal under anaesthesia Intestinal obstruction managed by gastrostomy Perirenal abscess managed by open drainage
4a	Bleeding (hypovolaemic shock) requiring ICU management Adult respiratory distress syndrome requiring ICU management Hyposaturation requiring ICU management Pulmonary oedema requiring ICU management Heart failure requiring ICU management Hypothermia requiring ICU management Acute renal failure requiring ICU management Arrhythmias with haemodynamic instability requiring ICU management Severe atelectasis requiring intubation and requiring ICU management
4b	Urosepsis with multiple organ failure requiring ICU management
5	Any complication leading to death

12.2 Specific Complications in PCNL

12.2.1 Bleeding

Whilst bleeding remains a serious complication of percutaneous renal surgery, severe haemorrhage is now relatively rare, with approximately only 2.5–3.8% of cases requiring blood transfusion [7]. Approximately 1% of these patients may require radiological intervention such as selective arterial embolization and in current practice the need for nephrectomy for uncontrolled bleeding is less than 1 in 1000 cases [8]. Bleeding from parenchymal vessels is commonly encountered during tract dilation, and this is usually well controlled by tamponade from the nephrostomy tube placed at the end of the procedure. There is no evidence that either balloon or serial dilation is safer, and either method is acceptable. Dilatation be it with single step, serial metal dilation, i.e. Alken telescopic rod system or a balloon tract dilator is a matter of personal choice. Ideal placement of the access tract is in Brodel's avascular plane, and in difficult cases deviation from this may cause heavier bleeding. Overaggressive torque application to the nephroscope or sheath may also tear vessels adjacent to the tract and cause bleeding.

If a bleeding vessel is seen in the tract, direct cautery may be attempted intraoperatively but this is rarely feasible. Most postoperative haemorrhage can be safely managed by clamping the nephrostomy and delaying removal. Compression dressings over the puncture site may also help. Regular close monitoring of these patients is essential to confirm that these conservative measures are proving effective. Early irrigation of the nephrostomy is not advised, as this may dislodge clot that is forming and perpetuate bleeding.

Severe or ongoing haemorrhage, particularly from entry into a major vessel, requires prompt radiological intervention. Angiography followed by selective embolization is usually the management of choice, but endovascular stenting can also be performed in suitable cases and may preserve blood supply to the affected segment of kidney. A similar management strategy is appropriate for patients who present with delayed haemorrhage after discharge, as these are frequently due to pseudoaneurysm formation. Persistent haematomas may be drained percutaneously. Whilst rare, the urologist should always consider the need for emergency nephrectomy should radiological intervention fail or if uncontrollable haemorrhage occurs.

12.2.2 Damage to the Collecting System

The collecting system may be injured in a number of ways during the course of a PCNL. During the initial puncture and tract dilation, a "through and through" injury may occur, or misuse or misfiring of a lithotripter or laser can also cause direct damage. Tears may also occur from the use of excessive force or torque on the nephroscope and access sheath, causing avulsion of the PUJ or damage to the infundibulum.

Recognition of the injury is key to management. The procedure should not be continued as ongoing irrigation will lead to extravasation and increase the risk of infection. Stone fragments may also be washed out into the retroperitoneal space. Drainage of the collecting system is the key to management. A nephrostomy tube as well as a ureteric stent should be placed to optimize drainage. If significant extravasation of irrigant has already occurred, placement of a perinephric drain is also advised. If the injury is detected postoperatively, percutaneous placement of a drain under radiological guidance is wise. Depending on the extent and severity of the injury to the collecting system, these should be left from 3 to 14 days before performing a nephrostogram to evaluate healing of the collecting system. Care of these patients postoperatively would involve examination of abdominal signs such as abdominal guarding and watching for paralytic ileus.

In rare cases, ongoing urine leaks may require surgical reconstruction, in which case the opinion of an expert in the field should be sought. Complete avulsion of the PUJ is also an indication for reconstruction, which may be best done at the time of the injury as subsequent inflammation and scar tissue formation may make delayed reconstruction challenging. Long-term complications of damage to the collecting system include stricture formation and perirenal abscess formation.

12.2.3 Infection and Sepsis

Practically all large renal stones are colonized by bacteria, and unsurprisingly transient fever following PCNL is common, occurring in up to 30% of patients. Sepsis and septic shock are relatively rare, with rates under 1% [5]. All patients should have a preoperative urinalysis and culture before PCNL, and in the case of a positive culture appropriate antibiotic treatment is advised (24 h prior) to the procedure. Patients who have a prolonged procedure with high volumes of irrigant fluid used, and those with stones >20 mm in size are at higher risk for postoperative sepsis [9, 10]. A course of postoperative antibiotics may be appropriate in this group. In patients with obstruction of the renal tract from stones, midstream urine culture may not reflect infection in the proximal part of the tract. Culture of urine from the renal pelvis and stone sample culture should therefore be undertaken to ensure appropriate cover [11, 12]. While the choice of antibiotic should ideally be based on proven culture and sensitivities, where this is not possible treatment should be guided by local policy and resistance patterns, in conjunction with an assessment of the risk level of the patient.

Patients who do not respond appropriately to initial antibiotic treatment must be evaluated thoroughly for other potential sources of sepsis, and early imaging may be useful to rule out a urinoma or evolving perirenal abscess requiring drainage. Ongoing drainage of the urinary system is also essential, so stents and nephrostomies should be kept in until sepsis is well controlled. Close collaboration with colleagues from Critical Care, Microbiology and Radiology is essential.

12.2.4 Organ Injury

The bowel (predominantly colon but occasionally duodenum), pleura, spleen, and liver can all be injured during the course of PCNL access. This, however, is rare, with most series reporting a rate of organ injury of under 1% [3, 6]. The risk of bowel injury is significantly higher on left side, with thin, older patients being at particular risk. Other risk factors for bowel injury include prior intrabdominal surgery and horseshoe kidney. It has been suggested that the use of ultrasound may be superior to fluoroscopy in preventing bowel injury during PCNL [13].

Extraperitoneal bowel injuries can frequently be managed conservatively without the need for surgical exploration [3]. Care should be taken to leave a large bore nephrostomy tube in situ. The communication between the kidney and bowel must be separated, and at the time of tube drain removal the nephrostomy tube should be pulled back into the retroperitoneal space and then removed. Drainage of the collecting system can be achieved with insertion of a ureteric stent. Intravenous antibiotics should be commenced for a minimum of 7 days. If a colocutaneous fistula forms, temporary defunctioning with a colostomy or ileostomy may be required. Intraperitoneal injuries usually require exploration and repair with a washout of the contaminated peritoneal cavity.

Pleural injuries are relatively rare with lower pole punctures but the risk increases substantially with supra-11th rib punctures to as high as 35% [14]. Performing the initial puncture in full expiration and the use of ultrasound or CT to visualize the pleura have been suggested as methods of reducing this risk. Placement of a chest drain is usually sufficient to allow resolution of a haemo or pneumothorax but in rare cases thoracoscopy and thoracotomy have been reported.

Injuries to the liver and spleen are thankfully uncommon but may have catastrophic consequences. Significant injuries during the course of access may require immediate open exploration for haemostasis. Injuries not apparent at the time of surgery can potentially be managed conservatively; however expert guidance should *always* be sought prior to embarking on this course of management.

12.2.5 Other Complications

PCNL has traditionally been performed in a prone position. This may present anaesthetic challenges, particularly in obese patients or those with cardiopulmonary disease. If care is not taken during positioning of the patient, there is the potential for nerve and pressure-related injuries during the course of a prolonged procedure. Modern positioning aids and supports may help to reduce the risk of these injuries. Supine PCNL is increasingly being performed and has comparable outcomes, with a similar complication rate [5].

Complications related to the use of irrigant can occur if adequate precautions are not observed. Cold irrigant may cause cause profound patient hypothermia and impair clotting. Use of cold irrigation fluids also lead to excessive shivering postoperatively so warming of the fluid (either by the use of an in-line heater or prewarmed bags) is essential [15]. Saline is the ideal choice of fluid, as glycine or water may be absorbed in large quantities through the tract and lead to hyponatremia. Care should be taken to minimize the entry of gas into the tract during irrigation as there have been reports of vascular air embolism as a consequence [16].

Steinstrasse ("stone street") occurs when multiple stone fragments pass into the distal ureter and cause obstruction. It can be prevented by the use of an occluding balloon catheter (Occluder™ Boston Scientific) in the renal pelvis or proximal ureter. This consists of a balloon with inflation channel and a guide wire and injecting port [17]. Other devices used are Accordion (R) (PercSys, Palo Alto, CA) which uses 2.9 Fr Hydrophilic coated device deployed retrogradely with an open-ended catheter [17].

Thermosensitive gels such as Backstop (™) can be used to prevent passage of fragments in the PUJ region and their subsequent passage in upper ureter [18].

When techniques such as "tubeless", mini and micro-PCNL are used, extraction of stone debris and fragments may be more challenging, and care must be taken to minimize the risk of distal migration of these fragments. Options for management include extracorporeal lithotripsy to the lead fragment, retrograde ureteroscopy, or repeat PCNL with antegrade ureteroscopy.

12.3 Prevention and Prediction of Complications

A good surgeon knows how to get out of trouble... a better one knows how to avoid it

It is increasingly understood that while complications in surgery are multifactorial, many of these factors can be identified and addressed ahead of time. While technique and surgical skill may minimize complications in an individual operation, changes in overall culture and practice are needed to reduce overall rates of complications. One major trend in recent years is subspecialization and the centralization of complex stone surgery such as PCNL at high-volume centres. There is a mounting body of evidence to suggest better outcomes as well as reduced complication rates in dedicated stone units. There is also evidence to suggest a reduced severity of complications with high-volume surgeons [19]. With increasing operative volume, it also becomes viable for a dedicated stone multi-disciplinary team meeting (MDT) to be held for preoperative planning and discussion. Access to support from other specialties such an interventional radiology and vascular surgery may also be better in larger units, so on the rare occasions when their support is required this may be more timely.

A key step in anticipating and avoiding complications in any surgical procedure is the use of the World Health Organization checklist (Fig. 12.1) [21]. A large, multicentre, international trial demonstrated that routine use of this simple checklist reduced not only complication rates but also overall mortality. This applied to hospitals in the developing world as well as in industrialized nations, across a wide range of surgical procedures. To increase relevance, the checklist can be adapted to specific procedures and local practice.

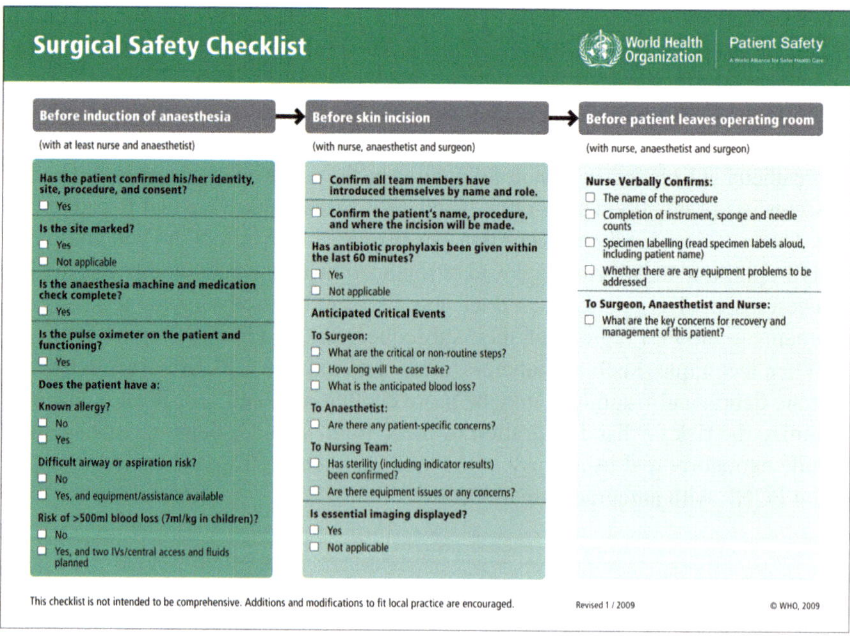

Surgical Safety Checklist

World Health Organization | Patient Safety

Before induction of anaesthesia → **Before skin incision** → **Before patient leaves operating room**

Before induction of anaesthesia
(with at least nurse and anaesthetist)

Has the patient confirmed his/her identity, site, procedure, and consent?
- ☐ Yes

Is the site marked?
- ☐ Yes
- ☐ Not applicable

Is the anaesthesia machine and medication check complete?
- ☐ Yes

Is the pulse oximeter on the patient and functioning?
- ☐ Yes

Does the patient have a:

Known allergy?
- ☐ No
- ☐ Yes

Difficult airway or aspiration risk?
- ☐ No
- ☐ Yes, and equipment/assistance available

Risk of >500ml blood loss (7ml/kg in children)?
- ☐ No
- ☐ Yes, and two IVs/central access and fluids planned

Before skin incision
(with nurse, anaesthetist and surgeon)

- ☐ **Confirm all team members have introduced themselves by name and role.**
- ☐ **Confirm the patient's name, procedure, and where the incision will be made.**

Has antibiotic prophylaxis been given within the last 60 minutes?
- ☐ Yes
- ☐ Not applicable

Anticipated Critical Events

To Surgeon:
- ☐ What are the critical or non-routine steps?
- ☐ How long will the case take?
- ☐ What is the anticipated blood loss?

To Anaesthetist:
- ☐ Are there any patient-specific concerns?

To Nursing Team:
- ☐ Has sterility (including indicator results) been confirmed?
- ☐ Are there equipment issues or any concerns?

Is essential imaging displayed?
- ☐ Yes
- ☐ Not applicable

Before patient leaves operating room
(with nurse, anaesthetist and surgeon)

Nurse Verbally Confirms:
- ☐ The name of the procedure
- ☐ Completion of instrument, sponge and needle counts
- ☐ Specimen labelling (read specimen labels aloud, including patient name)
- ☐ Whether there are any equipment problems to be addressed

To Surgeon, Anaesthetist and Nurse:
- ☐ What are the key concerns for recovery and management of this patient?

This checklist is not intended to be comprehensive. Additions and modifications to fit local practice are encouraged.

Revised 1 / 2009

© WHO, 2009

Fig. 12.1 WHO surgical safety checklist [20]

12.4 Identification of High-Risk Patients

It is increasingly recognized that certain patient groups are at higher risk of perioperative complications [22, 23]. The preponderance of these risk factors—in particular advanced age and metabolic syndrome—is increasing in most countries, posing additional challenges to the surgeon. One method of quantifying patient risk prior to major procedures is the use of scoring systems such as the Charlson Comorbidity Index. This has been shown to be useful in the context of PCNL, with higher scores correlating to higher rates of complications [24]. These may be used in conjunction with more detailed tests such as cardiopulmonary exercise (CPEX) testing to determine the risk of an individual patient for surgery, and to decide if surgical intervention is indeed the best management option. A summary of some factors that influence the risk of complications in PCNL follows in Table 12.3.

Table 12.3 Risk factors for complications in PCNL

Patient factors	Surgical/technical factors
Advanced age	Inexperienced/low-volume surgeon
High body mass index	Prolonged procedure
Abnormal anatomy e.g. horseshoe kidney	High irrigant volume use
Deranged clotting	Upper pole (supracostal) puncture
Large or staghorn stone	Multiple tracts/punctures
Diabetes mellitus	Excessive use of torque
Metabolic syndrome	Incorrect use of equipment
Hypertension	Bilateral procedure
Pre-existing renal failure	
Immunocompromise	
Urinary tract infection	
Transplant kidney	

12.5 Conclusion

While the overall risk of complications from PCNL has reduced dramatically in recent times, there is still room for improvement. Key strategies for reducing complication rates include identification and risk-stratification of challenging patients, close collaboration of the urologist with allied specialties such as anaesthesia, interventional radiology, and diligent compliance with safety measures such as the WHO checklist. Challenges for the future will include increasing rates of antibiotic resistance and an increasingly older patient cohort with more comorbidities.

References

1. Türk C, Petřík A, Sarica K, Seitz C, Skolarikos A, Straub M, Knoll T. EAU guidelines on interventional treatment for urolithiasis. Eur Urol. 2016;69(3):475–82.
2. Assimos D, Krambeck A, Miller NL, Monga M, Murad MH, Nelson CP, Pace KT, Pais VM, Pearle MS, Preminger GM, Razvi H. Surgical management of stones: American Urological Association/Endourological Society Guideline, PART II. J Urol. 2016;196:1161.
3. Michel MS, Trojan L, Rassweiler JJ. Complications in percutaneous nephrolithotomy. Eur Urol. 2007;51(4):899–906.
4. De la Rosette JJMCH, Zuazu JR, Tsakiris P, Elsakka AM, Zudaire JJ, Laguna MP, de Reijke TM. Prognostic factors and percutaneous nephrolithotomy morbidity: a multivariate analysis of a contemporary series using the Clavien classification. J Urol. 2008;180(6):2489–93.
5. Seitz C, Desai M, Häcker A, Hakenberg OW, Liatsikos E, Nagele U, Tolley D. Incidence, prevention, and management of complications following percutaneous nephrolitholapaxy. Eur Urol. 2012;61(1):146–58.
6. Dindo D, Demartines N, Clavien PA. Classification of surgical complications: a new proposal with evaluation in a cohort of 6336 patients and results of a survey. Ann Surg. 2004;240(2):205–13.
7. Armitage JN, Irving SO, Burgess NA, British Association of Urological Surgeons Section of Endourology. Percutaneous nephrolithotomy in the United Kingdom: results of a prospective data registry. Eur Urol. 2012;61(6):1188–93.
8. Keoghane SR, Cetti RJ, Rogers AE, Walmsley BH. Blood transfusion, embolisation and nephrectomy after percutaneous nephrolithotomy (PCNL). BJU Int. 2013;111(4):628–32.
9. Bootsma AJ, Pes MPL, Geerlings SE, Goossens A. Antibiotic prophylaxis in urologic procedures: a systematic review. Eur Urol. 2008;54(6):1270–86.
10. Lojanapiwat B, Kitirattrakarn P. Role of preoperative and intraoperative factors in mediating infection complication following percutaneous nephrolithotomy. Urol Int. 2011;86(4):448–52.
11. Mariappan P, Loong CW. Midstream urine culture and sensitivity test is a poor predictor of infected urine proximal to the obstructing ureteral stone or infected stones: a prospective clinical study. J Urol. 2004;171(6):2142–5.
12. Kulkarni CR, Subodh S, Date JA. Correlation between preoperative midstream urine culture, intra operative stone culture and intra operative renal pelvic urine culture with post operative fever in patients undergoing percutaneous nephrolithotomy (PCNL) for renal calculi. J Urol. 2020;203:e204. https://doi.org/10.1097/JU.0000000000000840.02.
13. Falahatkar S, Neiroomand H, Enshaei A, Kazemzadeh M, Allahkhah A, Jalili MF. Totally ultrasound versus fluoroscopically guided complete supine percutaneous nephrolithotripsy: a first report. J Endourol. 2010;24(9):1421–6.
14. Munver R, Delvecchio FC, Newman GE, Preminger GM. Critical analysis of supracostal access for percutaneous renal surgery. J Urol. 2001;166(4):1242–6.

15. Hosseini SR, Mohseni MG, Aghamir SMK, Rezaei H. Effect of irrigation solution temperature on complication of percutaneous nephrolithotomy: a randomized clinical trial. Urol J. 2019;16:525–9. https://doi.org/10.22037/uj.v0i0.4399.
16. Chahal D, Ruzhynsky V, McAuley I, Sweeney D, Sobkin P, Kinahan M, Gardiner R, Kinahan J. Paradoxical air embolism during percutaneous nephrolithotomy due to patent foramen ovale: case report. Can Urol Assoc J. 2015;9:E658–60. https://doi.org/10.5489/cuaj.2835.
17. Nakada SY, Pearle MS. Editors: Surgical management of urolithiasis: percutaneous, shock-wave and ureteroscopy. New York: Springer; 2013. p. 41.
18. Rane A, Bradoo A, Rao P, Shivde S, Elhilali M, Anidjar M, Pace K, John RD. The use of a novel reverse thermosensitive polymer to prevent ureteral stone retropulsion during intracorporeal lithotripsy: a randomized, controlled trial. J Urol. 2010;183:1417–21. https://doi.org/10.1016/j.juro.2009.12.023.
19. Opondo D, Tefekli A, Esen T, Labate G, Sangam K, De Lisa A, Shah H, De La Rosette J, CROES PCNL Study Group. Impact of case volumes on the outcomes of percutaneous nephrolithotomy. Eur Urol. 2012;62(6):1181–7.
20. World Health Organization. WHO guidelines for safe surgery: safe surgery saves lives. Geneva: World Health Organization; 2009.
21. Haynes AB, Weiser TG, Berry WR, Lipsitz SR, Breizat AHS, Dellinger EP, Herbosa T, Joseph S, Kibatala PL, Lapitan MCM, Merry AF. A surgical safety checklist to reduce morbidity and mortality in a global population. N Engl J Med. 2009;360(5):491–9.
22. Olvera-Posada D, Tailly T, Alenezi H, Violette PD, Nott L, Denstedt JD, Razvi H. Risk factors for postoperative complications of percutaneous nephrolithotomy at a tertiary referral center. J Urol. 2015;194(6):1646–51.
23. Turna B, Nazli O, Demiryoguran S, Mammadov R, Cal C. Percutaneous nephrolithotomy: variables that influence hemorrhage. Urology. 2007;69(4):603–7.
24. Unsal A, Resorlu B, Atmaca AF, Diri A, Goktug HNG, Can CE, Gok B, Tuygun C, Germiyonoglu C. Prediction of morbidity and mortality after percutaneous nephrolithotomy by using the Charlson Comorbidity Index. Urology. 2012;79(1):55–60.

PCNL: Bleeding Complications and Their Prevention

13

Rajesh Kukreja

Percutaneous renal surgery is associated with lower morbidity, but it is not without its complications. In a study by Lang et al. a multi-institutional survey of patients undergone PCNL, an overall complication rate was 26% [1]. The complication rates decreased from 61 to 3.7% with an increase in the level of experience [2]. Generally, the complications associated with PCNL are related to the puncturing of the pelvi-calyceal system. Besides the blood vessels of the kidney, the other structures which may be injured are the pleura, liver, spleen, lung, and colonic parts. This has been described in detail in chapter 12 by Rane et al.

Complications are generally related to the initial puncture with injury of renal blood vessels and the surrounding organs (e.g., pleura, colon, spleen, liver, lung). The Dindo-modified Clavien system [3] describes these (Table 13.1). Large studies comparing these rates of complications by Seitz et al. and Labate et al. reported that 4–5% of patients develop major complications (Clavien grade 3 or greater) [3, 4] (Table 13.2).

R. Kukreja (✉)
Urocare Hospital, Indore, India

S. R. Shivde (ed.), *Techniques in Percutaneous Renal Stone Surgery*,
https://doi.org/10.1007/978-981-19-9418-0_13

Table 13.1 Clavien–Dindo classification as applied to percutaneous renal surgery

Complication grade	Description
0	No complication
I	Deviation from the normal postoperative course without the need for intervention
II	Minor complications requiring pharmacological intervention, including blood transfusion and total parenteral nutrition
IIIa	Complications requiring surgical, endoscopic, or radiological intervention, but self-limited, without general anesthesia
IIIb	Complications requiring surgical, endoscopic radiological intervention, but self-limited, with general anesthesia
IVa	Life-threatening complications requiring intensive care unit management; single organ dysfunction, including dialysis
IVb	Life-threatening complications requiring intensive care unit management; multi-organ dysfunction
V	Death resulting from complications

Table 13.2 Showing comparison of complications of two series

		Clavien grade (complication %)					
Authors	Patient number	0	1	2	3	4	5
Seitz et al.	11,929	77	11	7	4.1	0.6	0.04
Labate et al.	5724	79	16		4.2		

13.1 Why Is There a Risk of Hemorrhage in PCNL?

Acute hemorrhage is the most common and most significant complication following percutaneous access into the upper urinary tract collecting system [5].

13.1.1 Pathophysiology of Bleeding Post PCNL

Let us take into consideration a few basic facts of the anatomy and physiology of the renal unit. Each renal unit is a high-flow arteriovenous network and receives 20% of the total cardiac output in each cardiac cycle. The vascular network of arteries and veins closely surrounds the collecting system. The source of bleeding during and after PCNL is the renal parenchyma. There is some inevitable bleeding from small peripheral arteries and veins and is generally not significant. The segmental and the interlobar vessels are the major vessels supplying the kidney and injury to these usually causes significant bleeding. The other factors responsible for bleeding are tract dilatation, intrarenal manipulations, and nephroscopy [5–9].

It is necessary to emphasize that an accurate puncture is the best way to minimize bleeding and related complications in percutaneous renal surgery.

How to make an ideal puncture?

1. It is always straight.
2. It traverses the shortest distance between skin as starting point and the center of the calyx as the end point.
3. It avoids the infundibular entry and the necks of calyces.

An inadvertent injury to the infundibulum leads to damage to interlobar artery (infundibular artery). The other significant cause of bleeding is resultant torque when access through an anterior calyx needs movement to visualize stones [5, 6].

The other factors responsible for intraoperative bleeding are use of tools such as wires, graspers, baskets, and lithotrites.

13.1.2 What are the Measures to Control/Contain Bleeding?

1. Use an access sheath of appropriate size
2. Use a nephrostomy tube postoperatively

Hemostasis is achieved by the collapse of the parenchyma onto itself. Please note that only the postoperative nephrostomy tube as large or larger than the sheath used during the surgery contributes to good hemostasis. The size of varying diameters has not shown to be significant in measure of blood loss postoperatively [10–12].

13.1.3 What are the Factors Affecting Blood Loss?

The CROES PCNL study details many of these factors [13].

The most important factors are

1. Larger access sheath size
2. Prolonged operative time
3. Case load/center volume (low, mid, high)
4. Stone burden
5. Multiple tracts
6. Loss of percutaneous tract
7. Pelvicalyceal tears and manipulations of instruments

The other factors responsible are patient characteristics, renal pelvic perforations, supracostal punctures. The technical factors responsible for upper calyx puncture bleeding are the longer length of the tract and the obliquity. The skin puncture remains inferior to the punctured calyx even if a supracostal puncture is made [5–9]. Changing the direction of the tract to reach the renal pelvis may result in injury to the adjacent parenchyma with its vascular supply. It is advisable to enter the upper calyx through a straight and direct tract in line with the upper infundibulum and pelvis.

Technical complications such as the pelvic perforations and loss of access lead to excessive bleeding. **It is very strongly advised to stage the procedure**. When dealing with complex calculi with significant stone burden staging allows the injury to heal and reduce the blood loss [6]. Loss of percutaneous access can lead to loss of tract tamponade and uncontrolled bleeding from the renal parenchyma. **It should be a standard protocol to use initial guide and safety wires** to avoid loss of access.

13.2 Clinical Presentation in Cases of Bleeding Following PCNL

About 24% of cases present within 24 h [14]. Kessaris et al. reported a bleeding in 0.8% of cases in a series of 2200 patients. Delayed bleeding (41%) presented between 2 and 7 days after surgery, and 35% presented more than 7 days later.

13.3 Fate of Intraoperative and Perioperative Bleeding

13.3.1 Venous Bleeding

It is generally self-limiting and does not lead to hemodynamic instability. Remedial measures include maneuvers such as proper positioning of the Amplatz sheath. These methods tamponade the bleeding vessel. The other measure is to increase the pressure of the irrigating fluid to overcome the bleeding. This may lead to fluid absorption and a condition like TUR syndrome. A watchful anesthetist would notice an increase in diastolic pressure and hence an increase in central venous pressure. This should be aggressively managed using diuretics and management in postoperative ITU unit.

13.3.2 Arterial Bleeding

A significant arterial bleeding is identified by a fall in blood pressure, hemodynamic instability, and poor vision. This should necessitate stopping and staging the procedure.

A significant bleeding presents in many ways such as bleeding through and around the nephrostomy tube, clots in the bladder with clot retention, hemodynamic instability (fall in blood pressure, tachycardia, fall in urine output). Development of perinephric hematoma and hypovolemic shock are late signs of slow and steady bleeding and should be managed aggressively. A constant dialogue between surgical and anesthesia team avoids further morbidity.

13.4 Algorithm for the Management of Intraoperative Bleeding

13.4.1 Postoperative Hemorrhage

Factors responsible for postoperative hemorrhage

1. Strenuous activity
2. Infections
3. Preoperative and postoperative anti-coagulant therapy

The incidence of this bleeding is 1% as reported by Seitz et al. in a large series of 11,929 cases. They needed active treatment in 0.4% of cases [3].

13.4.2 Pathophysiology of Delayed Hemorrhage

It is usually a result of arteriovenous fistulas or arterial pseudoaneurysms, with the latter being more common.

The lacerated artery is a high-pressure system and will leak into a lower pressure system: a vein (fistula) or the parenchyma or hilar areolar tissue (pseudoaneurysm).

Arteriovenous fistulae occur when a paired set of artery and vein is injured, and arterial blood enters directly into the vein. The weak vein wall cannot sustain the high arterial pressure and ruptures. Bleeding into the collecting system is most noted, but it can be outside the kidney as well. The latter should be suspected if the hematocrit falls but the urine remains relatively clear. It can be confirmed with contrast CT scan with CT angiography or ultrasonography with Doppler.

An arterial pseudoaneurysm occurs when an artery is injured, clots off, and then intermittently ruptures, often clotting off again at variable intervals. Continuous bleeding suggests an arteriovenous fistula, and intermittent bleeding suggests arterial pseudoaneurysm, but the distinction is not critical because treatment is the same.

As soon as patient reports fresh bleeding, patient should be advised indoor admission and an urgent angiography which is diagnostic as well as therapeutic [14].

Richstone et al. reported series of 57 patients undergoing angiography in their data of 4695 percutaneous renal surgeries [15]. The commonest findings were renal pseudoaneurysms (47%). They observed contrast extravasation from a lacerated renal vessel in (22%) of cases. Arteriovenous fistulae were seen in (22%) of cases. Renal arterial dissection was seen in two patients and one instance each of a hypervascular area, a vascular "cut-off" sign. 17.5% patients had more than one lesion. The risk factors identified in these cases were staghorn calculi and multiple tracts. It is difficult to diagnose venous injuries by angiography as these situations present without demonstrable findings. Luckily venous origin usually responds well to conservative management.

The standard treatment of renal arteriovenous fistulae and arterial pseudoaneurysms is selective angioembolization, which is highly effective.

13.4.3 Management

The flowchart bellow (Fig. 13.1) gives a broad guideline to approach and manage intraoperative bleeding.

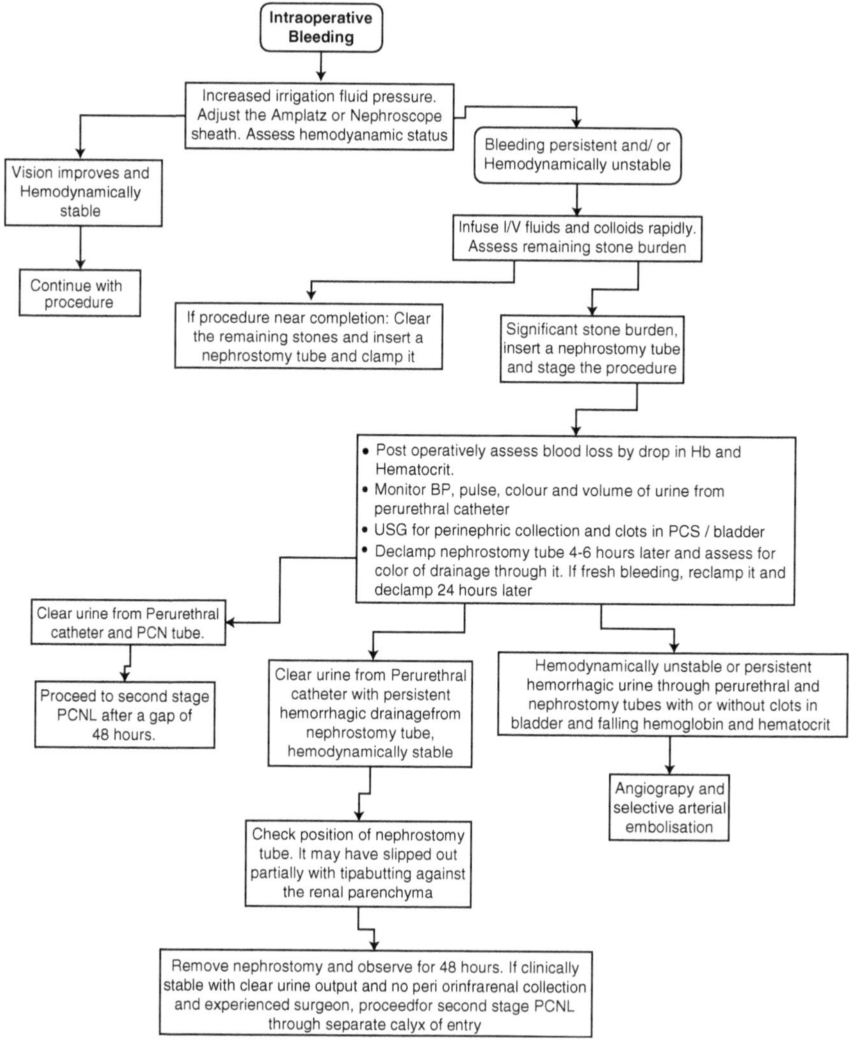

Fig. 13.1 Showing management of intraoperative or postoperative persistent bleeding

13.4.4 How Do You Manage Venous Hemorrhage During PCNL?

Commonly, intraoperative bleeding during PCNL is venous in origin

1. Increase the irrigating fluid pressure and
2. The placement of Amplatz sheaths: this step usually tamponades parenchymal bleeding and allows the urologist to continue the procedure

13.4.5 What To Do If Placement of the Sheath and Removal of Clots Does Not Restore Vision?

It is strongly advised to place and clamp a large (20–24 Fr) re-entry nephrostomy tube. This step facilitates clotting and hemostasis [6, 16]. Staging the procedure in such cases allows the injury to heal and reduces the blood loss at a subsequent stage [6]. The second stage surgery should be planned once the patient is hemodynamically stable with clear urine from the nephrostomy tube and per urethral catheter and after a minimum of 48 h delay.

- Minimal tract dilatation and limiting the procedure time help in limiting the renal trauma.
- If hemorrhage continues, Kaye tamponade balloon catheter can be inflated in the renal parenchyma to tamponade the venous bleeding. This 36 F occlusive balloon is inserted over a 5 F ureteral stent. It has an internal 14 F lumen that allows drainage of the renal pelvis. The Kaye catheter tamponades the nephrostomy tract and also drains the renal pelvis [16].
- A regular close monitoring is advised in the postoperative period. Pulse and blood pressure assessment with monitoring of urine output and urine and drain colour (both in the drain bag and urethral catheter bag) is done at regular intervals. A drop in hemoglobin and change in hematocrit mandate stepping up of treatment as per algorithm in Fig. 13.1.

Periodic ultrasonography is done to assess presence of pelvicalyceal or perinephric clots and collections.

After stabilization with crystalloids and blood products, patients should undergo renal angiography and super selective embolization. The rate of postoperative hemorrhage necessitating angioembolization has been reported at 0.8–1.3% [14, 15]. In a series of 4695 patients who underwent PCNL for various indications, Richstone and colleagues reported that 1.2% of patients postoperatively needed angioembolization [15].

In a multi-institutional review of 10 sites, renal angioembolization as a therapeutic intervention in the management of renal trauma had a success rate of 90% [17].

13.4.6 Indications for Angiography

1. Gross hematuria with clots
2. Decreasing hematocrit that does not respond to conservative management

3. Persistent/recurrent hypotension
4. Bleeding through nephrostomy
5. Clots in bladder/perinephric growing hematoma
6. Failed conservative treatment
7. Hemorrhagic shock

13.4.7 Complications of Angiography and Selective Angioembolization

1. There is a risk of arterial dissection, arterial perforation, and "non target" embolization. Nontarget embolization can occur with migration of the embolization medium, such as alcohol, coils, gel foam, glue, or particles [17]
2. Post-infarction syndrome: this includes flank pain, nausea, and vomiting. It is seen in majority of the patients. Fortunately, it is self-limiting
3. Contrast Induced Nephropathy (CIN)
4. Embolization induced loss of renal parenchyma
5. Allergy or hypersensitivity to contrast agents

CIN is directly related to the amount of contrast injected. Risk factors include diabetes and renal insufficiency. Preventive measures include intravenous hydration and *N*-Acetyl Cysteine (NAC) given in a dose 1.2 g twice a day prior and on the day of procedure [16].

In case the bleeding does not respond to selective embolization, a partial or total nephrectomy may be required [8].

13.4.8 Management of Perinephric Hematoma

The risk factors for post PCNL hematoma are
1. Preoperative ESWL
2. Patient on anticoagulation therapy

While a perinephric hematoma is a common finding post PCNL, a decreasing hematocrit despite a clear urine output should raise suspicion of a significant perinephric hematoma. An immediate or early ultrasound or CT scan diagnoses the problem. If conservative measures fail, then renal angiography and super selective embolization should be performed to identify and embolize the bleeding arterial branches. A percutaneous drain could be placed after the hematoma liquifies.

13.5 Role of Medical Therapy in Preventing or Reducing Hemorrhage Following PCNL

13.5.1 Tranexamic Acid

Tranexamic acid is a synthetic derivative of the amino acid lysine. It has strong affinity for 5 lysine binding sites of plasminogen. It acts as an antifibrinolytic. It competitively inhibits the activation of plasminogen to plasmin. Plasmin molecule is responsible for the degradation of fibrin. Fibrin is the basic framework for the formation of blood clot during hemostasis.

Kumar and colleagues demonstrated reduced blood loss, reduced transfusion rate and reduced operative time in patients receiving tranexamic acid. They followed the protocol of 1 g tranexamic acid at induction followed by 3 oral doses of 500 mg for 24 h [18].

The safety of routine use of tranexamic acid in surgical patients remains uncertain. A modest increase in the risk of thromboembolic effects could outweigh the benefits of reduced blood use [19]. There have been some promising reports of use of tranexamic acid in trauma patients. These have shown significant reduction of mortality and no significant risk of thromboembolic events in the said CRASH-2 study. The patients who had tranexamic acid also showed significantly reduced risk of myocardial infarction. Although some increased risk might be expected on theoretical grounds, recent evidence from the CRASH-2 (Clinical Randomization of an Antifibrinolytic in Significant Hemorrhage) appears to be encouraging [20, 21]. More studies are needed to evaluate the use of such agents in bleeding episode after PCNL.

References

1. Lang EK. Percutaneous nephrostolithotomy and lithotripsy: a multi institutional survey of complications. Radiology. 1987;162:25–30.
2. Duvdevani M, Razvi H, Sofer M, et al. Third prize: contemporary percutaneous nephrolithotripsy: 1585 procedures in 1338 consecutive patients. J Endourol. 2007;21:824–9.
3. Seitz C, Desai M, Häcker A, et al. Incidence, prevention, and management of complications following percutaneous nephrolitholapaxy. Eur Urol. 2012;61:146–58.
4. Labate G, Modi P, Timoney A, et al. The percutaneous nephrolithotomy global study: classification of complications. J Endourol. 2011;25:1275–80.
5. Wolf JS. Percutaneous approaches to the upper urinary tract collecting system. In: Campbell-Walsh urology. 11th ed. Amsterdam: Elsevier; 2012.
6. Kukreja R, Desai M, Patel S, et al. Factors affecting blood loss during percutaneous nephrolithotomy: prospective study. J Endourol. 2004;18:715–22.
7. Stoller ML, Wolf JS, St Lezin MA. Estimated blood loss and transfusion rates associated with percutaneous nephrolithotomy. J Urol. 1994;152:1977.
8. Keoghane SR, Cetti RJ, Rogers AE, et al. Blood transfusion, embolisation and nephrectomy after percutaneous nephrolithotomy (PCNL). BJU Int. 2012;111:628–32.
9. El-Nahas AR, Shokeir AA, et al. Post-percutaneous nephrolithotomy extensive hemorrhage: a study of risk factors. J Urol. 2007;177:576.
10. Lu Y, Ping JG, Zhao XJ, et al. Randomized prospective trial of tubeless versus conventional minimally invasive percutaneous nephrolithotomy. World J Urol. 2013;31:1303–7.
11. Maheshwari PN, Andankar MG, Bansal M. Nephrostomy tube after percutaneous nephrolithotomy: large bore or pigtail catheter? J Endourol. 2000;14:735–7.
12. Desai MR, Kukreja R, Desai MM, et al. A prospective randomized comparison of type of nephrostomy drainage following percutaneous nephrostolithotomy: large bore versus small bore versus tubeless. J Urol. 2004;172:565–7.
13. Yamaguchi A, Skolarikos A, Buchholz NP, et al. Operating times and bleeding complications in percutaneous nephrolithotomy: a comparison of tract dilation methods in 5537 patients in the Clinical Research Office of the Endourological Society Percutaneous Nephrolithotomy Global Study. J Endourol. 2011;25:933–9.

14. Kessaris DN, Bellman GC, Pardalidis NP, et al. Management of hemorrhage after percutaneous renal surgery. J Urol. 1995;153:604–8.
15. Richstone L, Reggio E, Ost MC, et al. Hemorrhage following percutaneous renal surgery: characterization of angiographic findings. J Endourol. 2008;22:1129–35.
16. Ardeshir R, Smith AD, Siegel DN, eta l. Management of hemorrhagic complications associated with percutaneous nephrolithotomy. J Endourol. 2009;23:1763–7.
17. Breyer BN, McAninch JW, Elliott SP, Master VA. Minimally invasive endovascular techniques to treat acute renal hemorrhage. J Urol. 2008;179:2248–53.
18. Kumar S, Singh SK, et al. Tranexamic acid reduces blood loss during percutaneous nephrolithotomy: a prospective randomized controlled study. J Urol. 2013;189(5):1757–61.
19. Ker K, Edwards P, et al. Effect of tranexamic acid on surgical bleeding: systematic review and cumulative meta-analysis. BMJ. 2012;344:e3054.
20. The CRASH-2 Collaborators. Effects of tranexamic acid on death, vascular occlusive events, and blood transfusion in trauma patients with significant hemorrhage (CRASH-2): a randomized, placebo-controlled trial. Lancet. 2010;376:23–32.
21. Myles PS, Smith J, Knight J, Cooper DJ, Silbert B, McNeil J, et al. Aspirin and tranexamic acid for coronary artery surgery (ATACAS) trial: rationale and design. Am Heart J. 2008;155:224–30.

Exit Strategies for PCNL

14

Pankaj N. Maheshwari

14.1 Introduction

Placement of the post-procedure nephrostomy tube is one of the important steps of the PCNL that would impact the post-operative course and morbidity to the patient. For a long-time nephrostomy tube of the size just smaller than the size of the nephrostomy tract was placed at the end of the procedure. This was done with an intent to aid haemostasis, drain purulent material or blood clots, and provide future renal access whenever needed.

14.2 Options

Placement of the nephrostomy tube has been a standard of care for many years. The teaching was to place a tube that is about 2–4 Fr smaller than the access tract. The options for post-PCNL drainage have been a nephrostomy tube or nephroureteral stent, an internal or ureteral stent, or no drainage tube at all, i.e. tubeless procedure [1–5]. Over the last one-and-a-half decade, the thinking about the need and the size of the nephrostomy tube had evolved and changed [1, 4–6].

14.2.1 Is the Size of the Nephrostomy Tube Important?

We have moved a long way from large bore nephrostomy tube to the placement of no tube at all. This change was brought about by the observation that presence of a

P. N. Maheshwari (✉)
Fortis Hospital, Mumbai, India

S. R. Shivde (ed.), *Techniques in Percutaneous Renal Stone Surgery*,
https://doi.org/10.1007/978-981-19-9418-0_14

large bore nephrostomy tube caused significant post-operative pain and led to prolonged post-nephrostomy tube removal leak and bleeding. Our group published the first study that showed that the size of the nephrostomy tube could be reduced from the conventional 28 Fr (after a 30 Fr tract) to a 9 Fr pigtail catheter [7]. There was no increase in bleeding rates, tract healed faster hence less leak, pain was significantly less, and the access was still maintained. After this study from our unit multiple studies validated our claim [1, 8, 9] leading to an attempt to completely stop using the nephrostomy tube- the "tube-less PCNL" [2, 3].

14.2.2 Is Nephrostomy Tube Needed for Haemostasis?

Bleeding is the most dreaded complication during PCNL. The major source of bleeding is bleeding from the parenchyma, infundibulum, or the tract. The tract starts from skin, goes via the abdominal musculature and enters the renal parenchyma till the calyx. Skin and musculature bleeding is never significant and is easy to control. It is the parenchymal bleeding that bothers us. It is shown that the bleeding would reduce or stop once the tract collapses. It does not need a tamponade of a nephrostomy tube [10].

14.2.3 Is Nephrostomy Needed for Drainage?

It is an established fact that the nephrostomy tube provides the best drainage of the collecting system hence it would be of an advantage if the bleeding during the procedure is significant but, in a patient, where the bleeding is minimal, even a ureteral stent would drain equally well [6, 11].

In another scenario of infected hydronephrosis with calculus, nephrostomy tube would help better drainage of the purulent urine and would also serve as an access for second stage (as the procedure would get staged because of infection or unexpected pyonephrosis).

In the event of a large perforation in the pelvicalyceal system (PCS) during the PCNL, placement of a large drainage tube would be vital.

14.2.4 Types of Nephrostomy Tubes

Malecot Catheter Placed with or without its wings. Advantages: good drainage, cheap and self retaining.

Balloon Catheter Routine urethral Foley used. Problems: balloon would be large and obstructive for some systems, still needs a skin suture for fixation.

Pigtail Catheter Easily available, self-retaining, reduced leak, less pain.

Cope Catheter Like a pigtail catheter but with a better retention mechanism. Not easily available.

Nephroureteral Stent Has a renal drainage segment and continues down the ureter as a ureteral stent. Gives an excellent control over the entire collecting system without the risk of dislodgement.

Circle Catheter Most secure system but needs two percutaneous accesses. No place in today's practice.

14.2.5 Tubeless PCNL

This idea of PCNL without a nephrostomy tube was initially proposed by Wickham in 1984, but was refuted by Winfield in 1986 reporting disastrous complications. It was later revived almost a decade later by Bellman in 1997. Tubeless generally means "no nephrostomy tube", some form of ureteral stent may be placed for a period of about 2 weeks. Tubeless PCNL has advantage with reduced pain and hence reduced need of post operative analgesics [1, 4, 12]. Patient does not need to carry an additional urine collection bag. The leak from the PCNL site is minimal hence reduced hospital stay. There is an early return to normal activities by the patient with a significantly reduced cost. The obvious disadvantage is that in the event of need for re-look nephroscopy, there is no access available. One should always consider this tubeless approach after careful consideration about the completeness of the primary procedure and stone free status.

Indications for tubeless procedure are cases where stone volume is moderate with resultant good stone clearance, uneventful procedure with the absence of bleeding.

Tubeless procedures are contraindicated in cases where we expect postoperative bleeding, in cases with operative findings of pyonephrosis, intraoperative pelvicalyceal system perforation and when we anticipate a second look staged procedure.

There are studies comparing tubeless versus small-sized nephrostomy tubes in patients undergoing PCNL [1, 5, 11].

14.2.6 Adjuncts to Tubeless PCNL

To reduce the risk of bleeding after tubeless PCNL, various adjuvant procedures have been tried. Mauracade et al. [6] reported electro-cauterization of the tract while Okeke et al. [13] attempted cryo-treatment of the tract. Both these methods are cumbersome and do not add much to the safety of PCNL. Apart from this instillation of haemostatic agents such as oxidized cellulose, gelatin sponge, and fibrin glue have been tried in the percutaneous tract [14–16]. At best it can be said that the utility and safety of these agents are uncertain, and they need further studies and evaluation.

14.3 Special Situations

14.3.1 Multiple Tracts

Making multiple tracts during PCNL for large volume stones and complex PCNL may be important for complete stone clearance [1]. It is not necessary to place nephrostomy tubes in every tract but due diligence should be exercised in choosing this strategy. Tube should be placed in at least one tract; either the major tract or the tract that has bleeding. This is important, in case a check nephroscopy is needed in these patients. Sizes for the chosen nephrostomy tube could vary from 8.5 to 34 Fr but a well-placed tube of any size, however, smaller would give an access in second look PCNL with equal ease [17].

14.3.2 Supracostal PCNL

Exit strategy after supracostal access entails multiple steps. Confirm that the pleura has not been violated. Place a nephrostomy tube if indicated and give an intercostal nerve block for analgesia.

Pleural integrity is confirmed by checking the Costo-Phrenic (CP) angle on fluoroscopy at the end of the procedure. If CP angle is clearly seen, there is unlikely to be a violation. If CP angle is obscured, aspirate the pleural fluid by puncturing it with the initial puncture needle. If the pleural fluid is clear, aspiration, placement of nephrostomy tube, and a DJ stent are all that is necessary. If the aspirate shows blood or purulent fluid then an additional pleural drainage tube is important [18].

14.3.3 Emergency Exit

Emergency exit during PCNL may sometimes be needed if there is a major bleeding or large pelvic perforation. It is prudent not to chase the fragments which migrate out of pelvicalyceal system after pelvic perforations as passage of instruments would make the perforations larger and more fluid extravasation would occur. One should always have a low threshold for stoppage of procedure when any of the above complication is noted or in case severe hemodynamic instability is observed. A constant dialogue with anesthesia team during difficult procedures helps safeguard the patient.

14.3.4 Bleeding

Try to assess the site of bleeding. Tract bleeding would usually stop once the Amplatz sheath is repositioned to tamponade the tract. Such bleeding usually stops on its own and may be better served by a large bore nephrostomy tube. If the bleeding from the tract is severe, tamponade can be achieved by a balloon catheter either a Foley or a Kaye's nephrostomy catheter. Once the nephrostomy tube is kept, clamp the nephrostomy tube and apply a compression dressing. Very rarely, if it is a single point arterial bleeder, electro-coagulation could be used.

Sometimes the bleeding could be from the opposite wall. This can happen due to the overshooting of the dilator during dilation of the tract. This bleeding will not stop just by insertion of the Amplatz sheath. It is important to take the Amplatz sheath beyond the bleeding site in the normal renal pelvis or upper calyx so that the nephrostomy tube can be placed across this bleeding site in the normal part of the PCS. Clamping the nephrostomy tube with a compression dressing will help in majority of cases.

In either situation, the patient is advised bed rest, hydrated well, covered well with antibiotics and if necessary, blood products could be replaced. A constant monitoring of vitals by the postoperative recovery team is strongly advised.

Management of bleeding following PCNL is discussed in Chap. 13.

14.3.5 Perforation

Large perforation of the PCS would make continuation of the procedure difficult. Extravasation of the irrigation fluid could lead to fluid overload. The collecting system would collapse making nephroscopy difficult. There is a risk of extrusion of the calculus fragments in the retroperitoneum. These extruded fragments can be a source of infection and a persistent worry for the patient.

Short duration procedure may continue with a small perforation but large perforations would need staging of the procedure. Keep the nephrostomy tube beyond the site of perforation. Also keep a DJ stent. Take care that the coil of the stent does not extrude outside the perforation. A postoperative PCN gram using contrast should be planned around day 3–7 to ensure healing and assess the status of residual fragments if any.

14.4 Summary

In summary, nephrostomy tubes and indwelling stents play a vital role in the exit strategy of all percutaneous procedures. Tubeless PCNL is an attractive option from the patient comfort point of view but to be recommended only if atraumatic access, no bleeding postoperatively, no perforation or suspected infection with complete stone clearance. We recommend placing a double J stent if the stone volume is large with resultant fragmentation, residual fragments, solitary kidney, and minor perforations of the PCS. A large bore PCN tube is indicated in scenarios involving infection, difficulties such as traumatic tract, perforations of the PCS, and bleeding. A small-bore pigtail nephrostomy tube would be considered in uneventful "Clean PCNL" with doubtful stone residue.

References

1. Desai MR, Kukreja RA, Desai MM, Mhaskar SS, Wani KA, Patel SH, Bapat SD. A prospective randomized comparison of type of nephrostomy drainage following percutaneous nephrostolithotomy: large bore versus small bore versus tubeless. J Urol. 2004;172(2):565–7.
2. Karami H, Jabbari M, Arbab AH. Tubeless percutaneous nephrolithotomy: 5 years of experience in 201 patients. J Endourol. 2007;21(12):1411–3.
3. Shah H, Khandkar A, Sodha H, Kharodawala S, Hegde S, Bansal M. Tubeless percutaneous nephrolithotomy: 3 years of experience with 454 patients. BJU Int. 2009;104(6):840–6.
4. Agrawal MS, Agrawal M, Gupta A, Bansal S, Yadav A, Goyal J. A randomized comparison of tubeless and standard percutaneous nephrolithotomy. J Endourol. 2008;22(3):439–42.
5. Choi M, Brusky J, Weaver J, Amantia M, Bellman GC. Randomized trial comparing modified tubeless percutaneous nephrolithotomy with tailed stent with percutaneous nephrostomy with small-bore tube. J Endourol. 2006;20(10):766–70.
6. Mouracade P, Spie R, Lang H, Jacqmin D, Saussine C. Tubeless percutaneous nephrolithotomy: what about replacing the double-J stent with a ureteral catheter? J Endourol. 2008;22(2):273–5.
7. Maheshwari PN, Andankar AG, Bansal M. Nephrostomy tube after PCNL: large bore or pigtail catheter? J Endourol. 2000;14(9):735–8.
8. Liatsikos EN, Hom D, Dinlenc CZ, Kapoor R, Alexianu M, Yohannes P, Smith AD. Tail stent versus re-entry tube: a randomized comparison after percutaneous stone extraction. Urology. 2002;59(1):15–9.
9. Pietrow PK, Auge BK, Lallas CD, Santa-Cruz RW, Newman GE, Albala DM, Preminger GM. Pain after percutaneous nephrolithotomy: impact of nephrostomy tube size. J Endourol. 2003 Aug;17(6):411–4.
10. Crook TJ, Lockyer CR, Keoghane SR, Walmsley BH. A randomized controlled trial of nephrostomy placement versus tubeless percutaneous nephrolithotomy. J Urol. 2008;180(2):612–4.
11. Shah HN, Sodha HS, Khandkar AA, Kharodawala S, Hegde SS, Bansal MB. A randomized trial evaluating type of nephrostomy drainage after percutaneous nephrolithotomy: small bore v tubeless. J Endourol. 2008;22(7):1433–9.
12. Feng MI, Tamaddon K, Mikhail A, Kaptein JS, Bellman GC. Prospective randomized study of various techniques of percutaneous nephrolithotomy. Urology. 2001;58(3):345–50.
13. Okeke Z, Andonian S, Srinivasan A, Shapiro E, Vanderbrink BA, Kavoussi LR, Smith AD. Cryotherapy of the nephrostomy tract: a novel technique to decrease the risk of hemorrhage after tubeless percutaneous renal surgery. J Endourol. 2009;23(3):417–20.
14. Aghamir SM, Khazaeli MH, Meisami A. Use of surgical for sealing nephrostomy tract after totally tubeless percutaneous nephrolithotomy. J Endourol. 2006;20(5):293–5.
15. Singh I, Singh A, Mittal G. Tubeless percutaneous nephrolithotomy: is it really less morbid? J Endourol. 2008;22(3):427–34.
16. Noller MW, Baughman SM, Morey AF, Auge BK. Fibrin sealant enables tubeless percutaneous stone surgery. J Urol. 2004;172(1):166–9.
17. Kim SC, Tinmouth WW, Kuo RL, Paterson RF, Lingeman JE. Using and choosing a nephrostomy tube after percutaneous nephrolithotomy for large or complex stone disease: a treatment strategy. J Endourol. 2005;19:348–52. https://doi.org/10.1089/.end.2005.19.348.
18. Maheshwari PN, Mane DA, Pathak AB. Management of pleural injury after percutaneous renal surgery. J Endourol. 1999;23(10):1796–72.

Residual Stones and Management 15

Subodh R. Shivde

15.1 Residual (Retained?) Fragments and Recurrent Stones Following PCNL

15.1.1 The Management and Postoperative Imaging Protocol

How does one measure the success or the efficacy of any stone treatment procedure? For a surgeon from the days of open surgery, it has been "complete removal of stones from a renal unit." From the perspective of a patient, it is the "complete removal of all stones/fragments" from the renal unit. The urology literature however sees it differently. It would quote various statistics such as Stone-Free (SF) rates, Clinically Significant (CS), and Clinically Insignificant Residual Fragments (CIRF). There is no uniformity as regards the various terminologies such as **residual**, **retained,** and **recurrent** stones in the context of percutaneous renal stone surgery or the method of reporting any of these. Worse still, there is no consensus as regards what criteria are to be used to define these and the imaging modality the urologists choose world over. In this chapter, let's look into this aspect of reporting of stone clearance rates and possible ways of prevention of residual stones in PCNL.

Routine postoperation imaging involves plain X-ray, ultrasonography, plain CT or non-contrast helical CT scan, contrast enhanced CT scan, and X-ray IVU to assess the stone-free status of patient. It would also involve a chest X-ray AP view to rule out accidental pneumothorax in case of higher or supracostal punctures. It would also be prudent to do nephrostogram in postoperative scenario with the

S. R. Shivde (✉)
Department of Urology, Deenanath Mangeshkar Hospital and Research Centre, Pune, Maharashtra, India

S. R. Shivde (ed.), *Techniques in Percutaneous Renal Stone Surgery*, https://doi.org/10.1007/978-981-19-9418-0_15

PCN (PerCutaneous Nephrostomy) tube in situ in special scenarios such as obstruction, urinary leak due to pelvicalyceal system rupture, and suspected residual fragments.

Historically stone treatment in the "Open Surgery Era" for the renal stones used postoperative imaging such as X-ray or ultrasound as imaging modalities and any stone fragments visualized during these tests would be called "Residual Fragments." In the modern era using PCNL, ureteroscopy, and shock wave lithotripsy, this definition of stone-free status has changed. Let us see how this concept of residual stones has evolved.

15.1.2 Residual Fragments (RF)

All and any fragments seen on imaging after 3 months of ESWL treatment is defined as Residual Fragments [1]. In the context of post PCNL scenario, any fragments remaining after surgery are considered Residual Fragments [2].

15.1.3 Clinically Insignificant Residual Fragments (CIRF)

These are stones seen on imaging modalities after surgery which are less than 4–5 mm, asymptomatic, non-infective stones [3–5].

15.1.4 Recurrent Stones

Recurrent stones as the term implies are the new stones formed in an operated patient where previous imaging had established stone-free status.

15.1.5 Postoperative Imaging Modalities

Let us now look at the ways to confirm presence or absence of stones in a postoperative scenario. Traditionally plain X-rays (X-ray KUB) and ultrasonography (USG KUB) have been used but in the modern era computerized tomography is now replacing the previous methods increasingly. These modalities have differing sensitivities for diagnosing residual stones [5]. Sensitivity of X-ray KUB ranges from 47.6 to 82%, USG 67.8%, and CT KUB being 89.2%. Sensitivity of CT scan would even be closer to 100% if UltraThin slice CT (UHCT) is used. Study by Raman et al. used these modalities after 30 days following PCNL to avoid seeing inconsequential dust of stones and overlapping shadows of JJ stents and nephrostomy tubes [5]. UHCT uses bone windows to differentiate between stones (<1600 HU) versus tubes (>1600 HU).

15.1.6 Residual Fragments Following PCNL and Their Fate

15.1.6.1 Why Do Stones Remain?

All current stone treatment modalities are aimed at breaking or pulverizing stone pieces. Increasing expertise has led the surgical fraternity to take on clearances of larger stone bulk, multiple stones, and even staghorn calculi. Fragmentation leads to multiplicity. Varying degrees of water or irrigant pressure leads to random movements of tiny stone fragments. Currently used telescopes with viewing degrees ranging from 0, 5, 15 and their rigid structure may miss the corners of the renal pelvicalyceal system and this will result in residual fragments. Add to these the hidden stones in areas such as diverticula, stones in location inaccessible to the viewing eye, i.e., posterior calyx entry, and anterior location of the stone and stones in horseshoe kidneys.

15.1.6.2 Consequences of the Residual Stones

1. They may lead to nothing—clinically insignificant [3].
2. These may grow leading to UTI (as in cases of struvite stones), hematuria, and microscopic or macroscopic nidus for a new stone formation.
3. Residual fragments may move or role over leading to clinical manifestation with resultant colic and morbidity. It is also a cause of repeated visits to hospital ER for pain management [6].
4. Last and not the least a source of perpetual anxiety for the patient and treating physician!

15.1.6.3 Why Do We Need to Watch the Residual Stones?

A study by Raman et al. [6] found that 40% of patients with residual fragments defined in this study by a criterion as less than 4 mm had a stone event, 57% of whom needed a surgical intervention. The study did a cost comparison between second look flexible nephroscopy versus expectant management of post PCNL residual fragments. The conclusion of the study was that observation was cost effective only for fragments smaller than 4 mm and not for fragments more than 4 mm. In another study by Raman et al. [5] considering 2 mm as residual fragment size, 43% of patients had a stone related event. They found time to recurrence to be 32 months. These would progress to stone growth, emergency room visit, need for hospitalization, or need for auxiliary procedures. Ganpule and Desai [2] in their study found that the most common site for post PCNL residual stones was the lower calyx. Renal pelvic stones had the best chance of clearance, i.e., stone-free status, provided the size was $<25\ mm^2$. Other predictors of persistence of residual fragments were renal failure, metabolic hyperactivity. They also stated that none of the patients with stone sizes $>100\ mm^2$ passed them spontaneously, conclusively proving the correlation between larger residual stone size and need for intervention. They also observed that spontaneous passage and clearance rate of residual stone following PCNL in their series (65.5%) were in accordance with stone-free rate of

CIRF after ESWL by Osman et al. [7] quoting a 78.6% rate without recurrence for 5 years. Ureteral fragments could pass spontaneously either by observation or good hydration with concomitant use of analgesics for colic with or without Medical Expulsion Therapy (MET) [8].

15.1.7 Prevention Strategies for the Residual Fragments

15.1.7.1 Pre-operation Planning

A thorough study of stone volume as regards size measurement and mapping of exact location preferably on CT KUB or CT IVU would help plan the PCNL procedure better. The need for extra punctures to reach abnormal location of outlier stones and identification of anatomical anomalies such as diverticular stones, malrotated renal units would help understand the complexity of the elective procedure.

Use of morphometry scores such as GUY'S and S.T.O.N.E. Morphometry would help patient counseling and also make realistic estimates of expected stone clearances [9–11]. This would result in better counseling of patients and make them aware of expected outcomes.

15.1.8 Intraoperative Measures

During surgery, measures such as thorough search inside the entire pelvicalyceal system in a systematic manner would allow us to obtain a visual clearance. This would be brought about by moving in the pelvicalyceal system from upper calyx, then to middle calyx if system allows and then through the lower part, each time visiting the PU junction to pick up any fragments moving around freely. A C-arm image would help corroborate the earlier confirmed visual clearance. In doubtful scenarios, if a rigid scope is unable to reach a particular location such as a calyx end, then a flexible nephroscope would be an invaluable tool [12, 13]. A final check could be made after withdrawing nephroscope leaving the Amplatz tube in situ to localize any debris or stone pieces. Angulating the Amplatz tube toward the so-called debris and reentering the system may help pick up some debris. An irrigation through the tube by saline washes using a Nelaton catheter or cut nasogastric tube will help clear fine particles at the end of surgery [14]. Although many centers prefer a "Tubeless" approach, we certainly recommend an indwelling JJ stent and a nephrostomy tube at the end of a successful PCNL.

A stent would allow the system to drain internally as well as help passage of stone debris keeping postoperative pain controlled. A nephrostomy would be useful for access in second look PCNL.

It is important to remember that not all stones are opaque on image intensifier and some small debris of stones could be missed as it is located behind the Amplatz tube (Fig. 15.1).

We advise gentle outward movement of scope and sheath simultaneously keeping in view the outermost extent of renal cortex. One generally encounters the stone

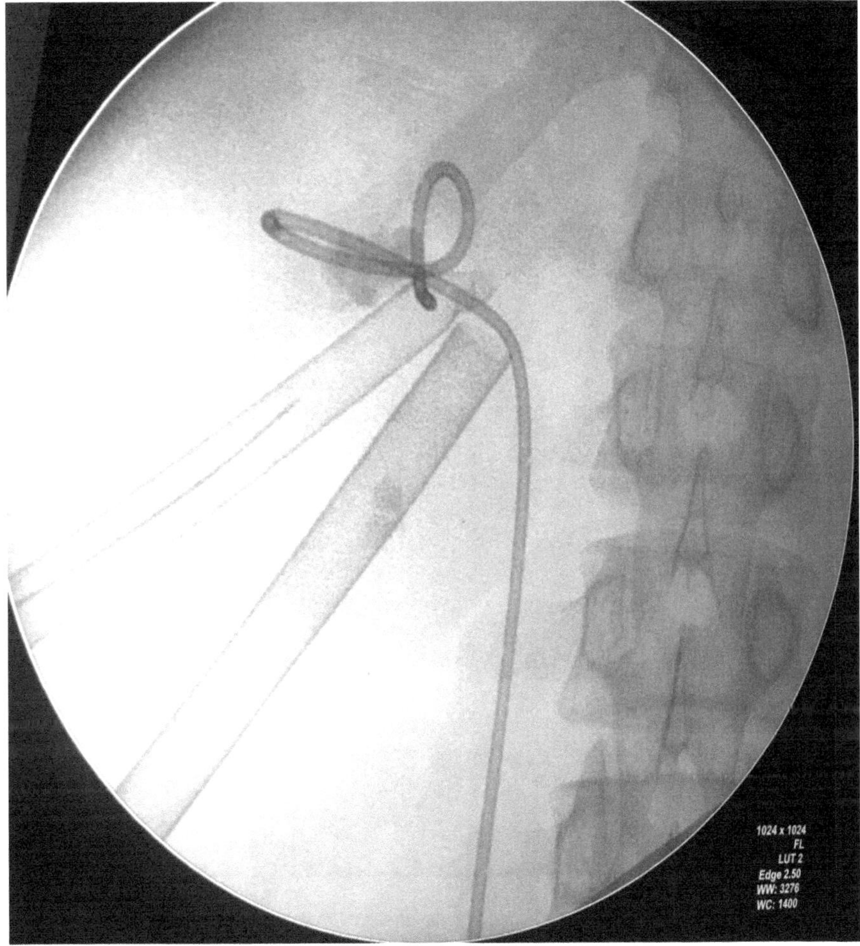

Fig. 15.1 Stone fragments seen behind the Amplatz sheath in the lower calyx

dust anteriorly, i.e., on the inferior aspect of telescopic vision assuming a normal posterior calyx puncture (Fig. 15.2).

Finally, we strongly recommend the use of flexible cystonephroscope to look for all possible stones or debris in order to get the best possible stone-free result.

15.1.9 Treatment of Residual Fragments

Now, if you have a scenario of residual stones, you may have to ascertain the volume of stone burden, it's exact location and plan after treatment

1. Small volume stone bulk <5 mm could be put for surveillance and wait till 30 days when patient due for stent removal. These patients would be suited for shock wave treatment with excellent results.

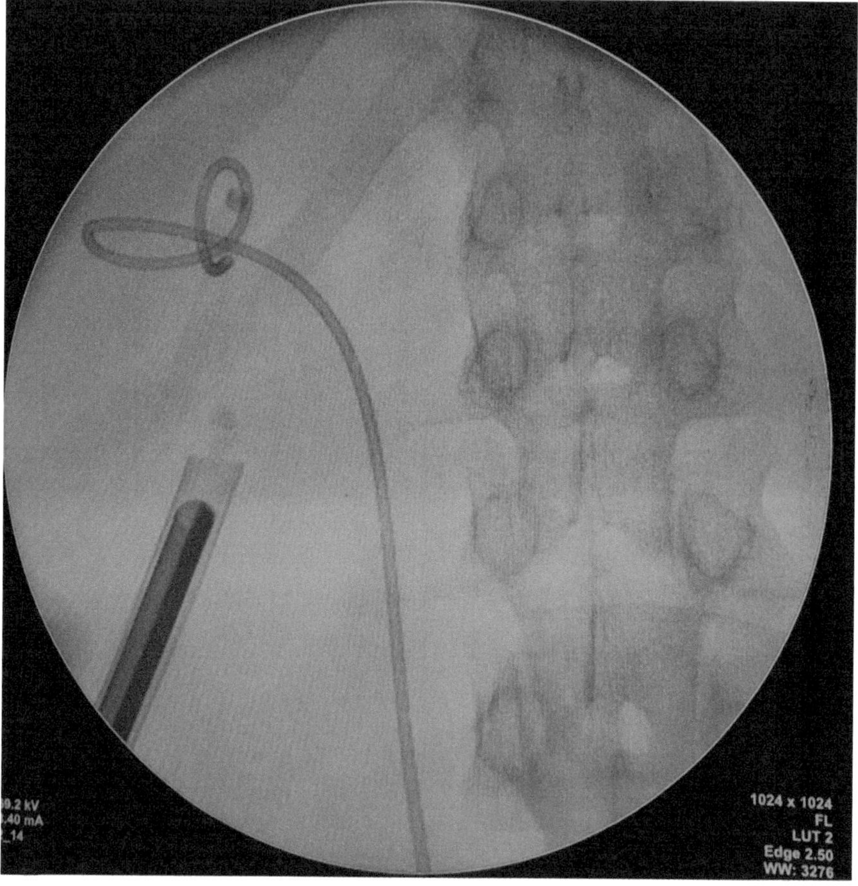

Fig. 15.2 Withdrawal of nephroscope and the sheath together to visualize stone debris

2. For larger stone bulk and multiple stones, a second look PCNL or flexible nephroscopy offers the best chance of achieving stone-free status. An effective stone-free rate of 97% has been reported. This would need second anesthetic and also result in additional cost [6].
3. Percutaneous chemolysis through PCN track using Suby G solution has been tried with varying success rates of up to 55.1% [15]. This study however documented 43.5% stone recurrence rate with a mean follow-up of 5.25 years.
4. Larger debris sizes >5 mm would qualify for sandwich therapy with options of shock wave followed by a secondary procedure such as RIRS. A retrospective comparative study with 2 groups matched for all variables including stone density, location of the stones, and the stone density measured as HU, Aminsharifi et al. [16] compared the stone-free rates in shock wave treated post PCNL patients with primary shock wave lithotripsy as treatment modalities. They

found a better stone-free rate in the post PCNL group as compared to primary shock wave group. Stone free being defined as no stone seen on non-contrast CT scan. Patients with stone HU < than 750 did significantly better than those with values above 750 HU.

All necessary steps in these scenarios would have to be carefully discussed with patients and alternative therapies would have to be given as options with pros and cons.

Further follow-up could be arranged with suitable imaging at regular intervals typically 3/6 monthly for the first year and then annually.

A dietary advice with medical therapies should be discussed with metabolic stone formers and recurrent stone formers to reduce chances of recurrence. A metabolic workup is indicated for recurrent stone formers and subsequent advice for drug therapy is a must.

A prophylactic antibiotic prescription would help all struvite stone formers, and this could be done taking into consideration the bacteriology and sensitivity patterns of urine, per operative pelvic fluid culture and the stone culture [17]. An interesting study results from our unit demonstrated the intuitive use of bacteriological study of PCN fluid and stone culture helping early identification of sepsis and swifter treatment commissioning using antibiotics smartly [12].

15.2 Review of Literature

Poulakis et al. used artificial neural networks to predict lower pole stone clearance after shock wave lithotripsy [18]. Their study predicted stone clearances with 92% accuracy. The pattern of dynamic urinary transport was the most influential predictor of stone clearances followed by measure of infundibulopelvic angle, body mass index, calyceal pelvic height, and stone size. Though not studied formally in a comparative scenario, residual fragments following PCNL could have the same fate as post ESWL stone fragments making all above factors significant.

Kacker et al. [19] evaluated the cost and outcomes for patients undergoing PCNL. They found out that larger stone burden independently predicted higher costs of surgery and lower stone-free rates ($p < 0.038$).

Choo and Jeong [20] in their study of 111 patients undergoing PCNL analyzed biochemistry of stone fragments. Patients were categorized based on the calcium phosphate content. The criteria set for stone-free status was fragments less than 2 mm on postoperative CT scan. They concluded that patients with more than 60% calcium phosphate content were significantly less likely to be stone-free making stone composition a crucial deciding factor for stone-free status.

Zhu et al. in their study used logistic regression model for predicting stone-free rate after minimally invasive PCNL. They concluded that increased stone number, size of the stone, location in calyx, staghorn calculus, and moderate to severe hydronephrosis were associated with decreased stone-free status [21, 22].

15.3 Conclusion

Nearly a third of published articles evaluating the outcomes of surgical treatments for renal stone disease do not define stone-free status. A wide variation exists in the use of imaging modality to detect residual stone burden. We need to have a standardized approach to reporting of the surgical outcomes following stone surgeries such as PCNL [13].

Non-contrast CT KUB with a defined criteria to quantify residual stone burden would be a good way forward, accepting the higher risk of dose of radiation compared to other modalities such as X-ray KUB and ultrasound.

A careful review of available images with a clear planning to target all stones and the so-called outliers will help achieve the elusive goal of stone-free status.

References

1. Lingeman JE, Newman D, Merton JH, et al. Extracorporeal shockwave lithotripsy: the Methodist Hospital of Indiana experience. J Urol. 1986;135:1131–4.
2. Ganpule A, Desai M. Fate of residual stones after percutaneous nephrolithotomy: a critical analysis. J Endourol. 2009;23:399–433.
3. Tan Y, Wong M. How significant are clinically insignificant fragments following lithotripsy? Curr Opin Urol. 2005;15:127–31.
4. Delvecchio FC, Preminger GM. Management of residual stones. Urol Clin N Am. 2000;27:347–54. https://doi.org/10.1016/S0094-0143(05)70263-9.
5. Raman JD, Bagrodia A, Gupta A, Bensalah K, Cadeddu JA, Lotan Y, Pearle MS. Natural history of residual fragments following percutaneous nephrostolithotomy. J Urol. 2009;181:1163–8. https://doi.org/10.1016/j.juro.2008.10.162.
6. Raman JD, Bagrodia A, Bensalah K, Pearle MS, Lotan Y. Residual fragments after percutaneous nephrolithotomy: cost comparison of immediate second look flexible nephroscopy versus expectant management. J Urol. 2010;183:188–93. https://doi.org/10.1016/j.juro.2009.08.135.
7. Osman MM, Alfano Y, Kamp S, Haecker A, Alken P, Michel MS, Knoll T. 5-Year-follow-up of patients with clinically insignificant residual fragments after extracorporeal shockwave lithotripsy. Eur Urol. 2005;47:860–4. https://doi.org/10.1016/j.eururo.2005.01.005.
8. De Coninck V, Antonelli J, Chew B, Patterson JM, Skolarikos A, Bultitude M. Medical expulsive therapy for urinary stones: future trends and knowledge gaps. Eur Urol. 2019;76:658–66. https://doi.org/10.1016/j.eururo.2019.07.053.
9. Thomas K, Smith NC, Hegarty N, Glass JM. The Guy's stone score—grading the complexity of percutaneous nephrolithotomy procedures. Urology. 2011;78:277–81. https://doi.org/10.1016/j.urology.2010.12.026.
10. Kanao K, Nakashima J, Nakagawa K, Asakura H, Miyajima A, Oya M, Ohigashi T, Murai M. Preoperative nomograms for predicting stone-free rate after extracorporeal shock wave lithotripsy. J Urol. 2006;176:1453–6. https://doi.org/10.1016/j.juro.2006.06.089.
11. Desai M, Sun Y, Buchholz N, Fuller A, Matsuda T, Matlaga B, Miller N, Bolton D, Alomar M, Ganpule A. Treatment selection for urolithiasis: percutaneous nephrolithotomy, ureteroscopy, shock wave lithotripsy, and active monitoring. World J Urol. 2017;35:1395–9. https://doi.org/10.1007/s00345-017-2030-8.
12. Kulkarni C, Shivde S, Date J, Patwardhan P. Mp15-02 correlation between pre-operative midstream urine culture, intra-operative stone culture and intra-operative renal pelvic urine culture with post-operative fever in patients undergoing percutaneous nephrolithotomy (PCNL) for renal calculi. J Urol. 2020;203(Supplement 4):e204.

13. Bagrodia A, Gupta A, Raman JD, et al. Predictors of cost and clinical outcomes for patients undergoing percutaneous nephrostolithotomy (PCNL). J Urol. 2009;181(4):490.
14. Panah A, Masood J, Zaman F, Papatsoris AG, El-Husseiny T, Buchholz N. A technique to flush out renal stone fragments during percutaneous nephrolithotomy. J Endourol. 2009;23(1):5–6. https://doi.org/10.1089/end.2008.0296.
15. Kachrilas S, Papatsoris A, Bach C, Bourdoumis A, Zaman F, Masood J, Buchholz N. The current role of percutaneous chemolysis in the management of urolithiasis: review and results. Urolithiasis. 2013;41:323–6. https://doi.org/10.1007/s00240-013-0575-6.
16. Aminsharifi A, Irani D, Amirzargar H. Shock wave lithotripsy is more effective for residual fragments after percutaneous nephrolithotomy than for primary stones of the same size: a matched pair cohort study. Curr Urol. 2018;12(1):27–32. https://doi.org/10.1159/000447227.
17. Steinberg PL, Hanover NH, Paris VM, et al. Evaluating "stone free status" in contemporary urologic literature. J Urol. 2009;181(4):490.
18. Poulakis V, Dahm P, Witzsch U, de Vries R, Remplik J, Becht E. Prediction of lower pole stone clearance after shock wave lithotripsy using an artificial neural network. J Urol. 2003;169:1250–6. https://doi.org/10.1097/01.ju.0000055624.65386.b9.
19. Kacker R, Meeks JJ, Zao L, et al. Decreased stone-free rates after percutaneous nephrolithotomy for high calcium phosphate composition kidney stones. J Urol. 2008;180:958–60.
20. Choo MS, Jeong CW. External validation and evaluation of reliability and validity of the S-ReSC scoring system to predict stone-free status after percutaneous nephrolithotomy. PLoS One. 2014;9(1):e83628. https://journals.plos.org/plosone/article?id=10.1371/journal.pone.0083628
21. Gücük A, Kemahlı E, Üyetürk U, Tuygun C, Yıldız M, Metin A. Routine flexible nephroscopy for percutaneous nephrolithotomy for renal stones with low density: a prospective, randomized study. J Urol. 2013;190(1):144–8.
22. Zhu Z, Wang S, Xi Q, Bai J, Yu X, Liu J. Logistic regression model for predicting stone-free rate after minimally invasive percutaneous nephrolithotomy. Urology. 2011;78:32–6. https://doi.org/10.1016/j.urology.2010.10.034.

Training for PCNL

16

Ashish V. Rawandale-Patil and Lokesh Patni

Percutaneous renal surgery as a treatment modality is continuously evolving, maintaining its association with its steep learning curve [1–3]. An image intensifier (II) or C-arm fluoroscopic imaging application and understanding of parallax techniques are essential prerequisites for performing percutaneous renal surgery (PCNL).

Several studies pertaining to training in PCNL have indicated that over 50 cases are needed to be done to acquire good skills and proficiency can be reached after about 100 cases [4–6].

An essential prerequisite to good percutaneous surgery is accurate access. It goes without saying that this cannot be obtained without a good knowledge of the anatomy of the kidney [7]. It is well known and well-published fact that difficult and multiple punctures lead to more morbidity and hence increase the complications such as bleeding, and damage to surrounding viscera [8]. Tract dilatation, intraoperative stone manipulation, exiting from the operative area and identification of an intraoperative error or complications also need a certain amount of learning. The management skills would only develop with repeated exposure to these varying scenarios.

Therefore, surgical training for percutaneous renal surgeries is an important facet of residency training and post-training proficiency.

A. V. Rawandale-Patil (✉) · L. Patni
Institute of Urology Dhule, Dhule, Maharashtra, India

S. R. Shivde (ed.), *Techniques in Percutaneous Renal Stone Surgery*,
https://doi.org/10.1007/978-981-19-9418-0_16

16.1 The Essentials of PCNL Training

Learning is the process of bringing a person to an agreed standard of proficiency through practice and instruction. Percutaneous renal surgery is no different from other surgeries.

Learning any new surgical art would include at least three distinct phases

Cognitive phase: Includes education of the anatomy and skillful use of instrumentation prior to performing a new psychomotor skill [9]. This phase of training is achieved by text reading, didactic lectures, instructional courses, illustrations and group discussions.

Integrative phase: Transferring the mental inventory of the steps into psychomotor action [10].

Autonomic phase: Undergoing sufficient repetitive practice so that the motor skills are executed automatically with very little cognitive input.

Conventionally there has been only one avenue for achieving the integrative and autonomic phase, namely in the operating room.

16.2 Operating Room Learning Opportunities

The **Halstedian** concept of **"see one, do one, teach one"** has been implemented for training surgical residents for many years. Recent practice trends have affected operating room training opportunities for the majority of surgeries including percutaneous renal surgeries. In continuation with the same PCNL training opportunities in the operating room have been marred by

1. Time constraints.
2. Financial pressures: to decrease the operating time and morbidity to keep the finances to a minimum.
3. Increasing complexity of cases at the tertiary centres which usually are the learning centres: making it mandatory for the senior consultant to operate the case.
4. Rapidly changing surgical technology posing a challenge to the trainer himself to learn the newer techniques.
5. Varied learning capabilities of the students: due to which a slow learner in the group would directly or indirectly slow down the learning of the group.
6. Medico-legal concerns in case of an untoward incident at the hands of the trainee or the trainer.

Unlike surgical procedures that involve the repetition of steps, each step of percutaneous renal surgery is typically performed only once per procedure except for a few steps like stone pulverization and retrieval. This limits the experience that can be gained during a single procedure. Also, the variability of each case, variations in surgical caseloads and variations in the practice trends amongst different centres leave gaps in training in specific key areas of percutaneous surgery.

Last but not least the trainee evaluation in the operating room involves subjectivity introduced by the teaching surgeon leading to the inclusion of significant biases.

"Gradual and progressive acquisition of skills in the operating room, after a period of observation by the student"—a classical style of teaching may not best suit PCNL. The trainee is unlikely to pass over the learning curve of PCNL during his training tenure.

Alternative training modalities, in the form of training sessions in the animal or simulation labs, are now being implemented. This potentially helps the trainees get over some part of their learning curve, increase the safety profile and get them ready to gain experience during their operating room training sessions.

The need for objectivity and the need to decrease subjectivity during surgical training and surgeon assessment is one of the few factors that have fueled the development of simulation for PCNL. This has given rise to the development of many PCNL simulation systems.

Simulation Maybe defined as an attempt to predict behaviour and response aspects of some naturally existing system by creating an approximate physical/mathematical/computer-aided model of it.

16.3 PCNL Simulation Today

Till date, we are devoid of the availability of a wholesome simulator. PCNL simulators of today are still finding their way and currently provide only part of the curriculum. They primarily provide training and not trainee assessment and tend to focus on the most difficult step of the learning curve, i.e. renal access.

The trainee, as well as the trainer, needs to know a few things about each other and the procedure before they start training and as they progress through the training period in order to make the most of the training period. It is important for the trainee to possess the required psychomotor skills for the PCNL. At the end of the training period, the trainee should know what to do, what not to do, how to do it, how to identify a mistake and rescue an unwanted situation.

The trainer needs to know how the trainee is progressing, and/or where they are on their learning curve and their progress in the psychomotor and cognitive skills.

Thus, certain prerequisites may be defined for a simulation program. A well-integrated and thought-out training curriculum needs to be planned.

A proposed 10-point schedule for a PCNL training curriculum today should include

1. Didactic teaching of retroperitoneal anatomy and 3-dimensional orientation of the kidney, pelvicalyceal system and the retroperitoneal organs
2. Instructions on the steps of PCNL
3. Defining and illustrating the common mistakes

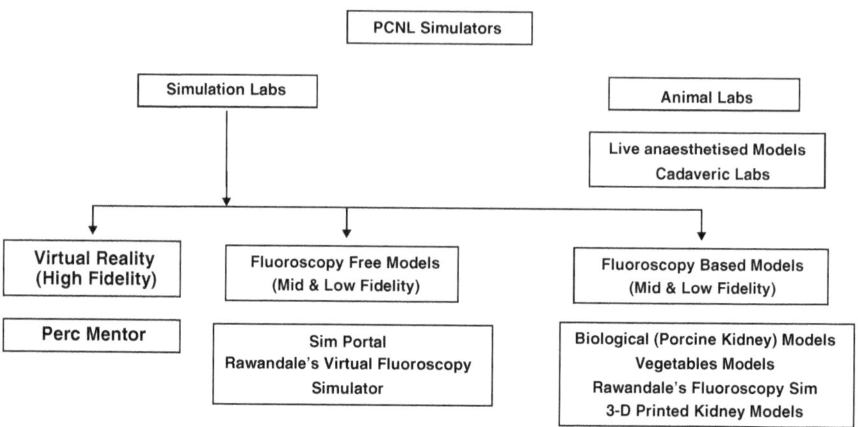

Fig. 16.1 Currently available training models

4. An initial and periodic evaluation to gauge the depth of perception of the trainee and assessment of the understanding
5. Skills training on a simulator
6. Provide immediate feedback when an error occurs
7. Provide feedback and suggestions for improvement at the completion of a trial
8. Opportunity to repeatedly train to perfection
9. Plotting the trainees' position on the "learning curve"
10. Tailor the training session as per the position of the trainee on the learning curve

The main challenge today remains to find the ideal simulator that can perform and fulfil all the above-mentioned requirements. Attempts are already underway in various parts of the world, some of which have surfaced in various publications and workshops. They broadly can be classified as in Fig. 16.1.

16.3.1 Animal Laboratory

Since the past, live animal models are being used extensively to develop new surgical techniques as well as train the novices of the art, to expand their skills. Animal models have distinct advantages over inert or nonbiologic bench models. They are more realistic to the live human scenario and are capable of providing almost human tissue-like haptic feedback as well as realistic bleeding and respiratory movements. Hence these scores are over the bench/inanimate models and are more appropriate as training and assessment tools. Live anaesthetized pig models are being used as practice models for PCNL. The porcine kidney replicates the human kidney to a good extent though it is more friable than the human kidney and has a less capacious pelvicalyceal system.

Animal labs have associated constraints. These are ethical concerns, animal rights issues, concerns about the spread of animal-borne diseases, animal availability, recurring cost, veterinary and anaesthesia assistance. These are some of the reasons for the high maintenance cost of animal labs. These constraints globally have been responsible for the preference of non-animal lab training avenues. Although the best, animal models cannot reproduce the human renal anatomy accurately. This has forced the medical fraternity and boosted the industry to look for alternative options to provide lab training opportunities for the trainees leading to a spurt in the development of PCNL simulators as a training tool.

16.3.2 Simulation Laboratory

In view of the pitfalls associated with animal labs, the inanimate simulation lab has established its prominent role in the training arena. Truly speaking, simulation labs are referred to setups with inanimate bench models of various fidelity. These models typically consist of a live human-like, torso and kidney. Various levels of simulations have been developed over the years, ranging from low-fidelity models to high-fidelity complex ones. In general, as the fidelity improves one would expect more realism during the simulation session. Another variation includes the hybrid/biological bench models which use animal organs along with an inanimate caricature/torso.

16.4 High-Fidelity Fluoroscopy Free Simulators

16.4.1 Why Are These Needed?

It is well known that a routine PCNL surgery exposes the operator to an X-ray time of approximately 7 min with a dose of about 110 mGy [16]. This led to the development of simulators which mimic fluoroscopy-like pictures to facilitate training also called computerized virtual-reality simulators. The PERC Mentor™ (Simbionix; Lod, Israel) uses tactile feedback, organ displacement with breathing, a virtual C-arm and mock instruments. A metal needle with a spatial sensor is used, and a contrast-filled digitally projected pelvicalyceal system is used for trial punctures. The fluoroscopic imaging is controlled by a foot pedal. Urine or fluid aspiration upon puncturing confirms an accurate puncture. The system also allows the passage of guide wires simulating the PCNL.

A trainee is exposed to various tasks of PCNL surgery such as understanding 3D anatomy, spatial orientation, tactile feedback using a virtual C-arm and angiographic instruments. A record is kept as regards operative time, the number of punctures, collecting system entries and record of errors can be kept. These come in handy for the instructors to appraise the trainee and monitor the progress of the structured environment. Training environment consists of a variety of incremental tasks and case scenarios. It teaches the user the fundamentals of 3D renal anatomy and surrounding structures. All endpoints, including overall operative time, number of punctures, fluoroscopy time, rib collisions, collecting system perforations, and blood-vessel injury, are recorded by the simulator and can be reviewed, allowing monitoring of the efforts of the trainees.

Animal models using the pigs have shown in phase I and II studies statistically significant improvement in the baseline performances of trainees [17, 18].

Disadvantages of PERC Mentor™ Though considered to be the top-line simulator with a high price tag; it comes with its inbuilt flip sides. The needle used for puncture is thick, has a wire emerging out of the hub and hampers movements. It lacks replication of tissue haptics and has a feel more like puncturing a slab of sponge. The sim has separate slots to pass wires and place catheters quite unlike an actual renal access procedure.

Computerization and software use brings their own disadvantages. Software hangs, pixelation of the needle, wire, etc. on the screen, dead ends/logically paradoxical ends with case scenarios. Virtual instruments on the screen move against the principles of physics. A limited armamentarium of instruments is available for use by the trainee.

16.4.2 Low- and Mid-Fidelity Simulators

16.4.2.1 Perc Trainer™

This is a commercially available low-fidelity PCNL trainer (Fig. 16.2). The features of this system are its ability to reproduce the ultrasound and fluoroscopic features of

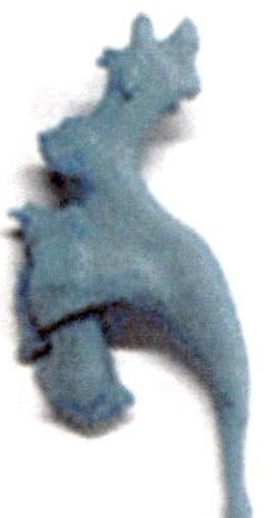

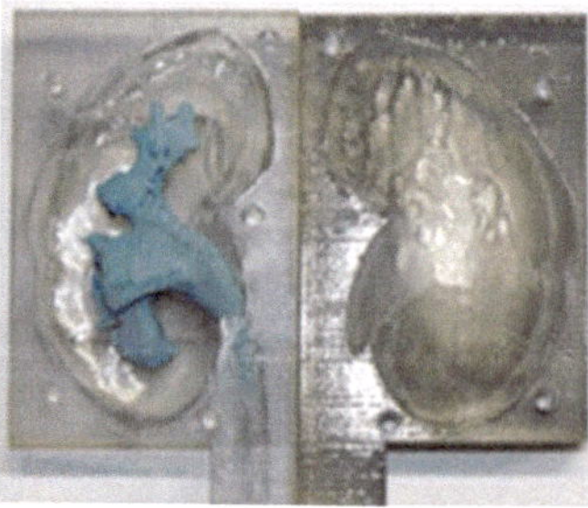

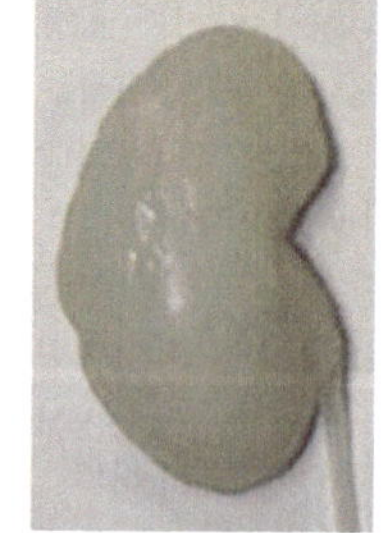

Fig. 16.2 Showing 3D printed models [3D Printed Kidney Model (Adams, F., Qiu, T., Mark, A. et al. Soft 3D-Printed Phantom of the Human Kidney with Collecting System. *Ann Biomed Eng* **45**, 963–972 (2017) https://doi.org/10.1007/s10439-016-1757-5, released under a Creative Commons Attribution 4.0 International License) [20]]

a real kidney. All the tasks of PCNL such as needle puncture, guide wire insertion, track dilatation, endoscopic inspection, stone fragmentation and retrieval are easily reproduced. The model can also be used in the supine position and can also be used for RIRS simulation.

The drawbacks of Perc Trainer™ are its cost and the need to replace the whole bench once damaged. It also uses real radiation causing hazards of radiation to the users.

16.4.3 3D Printed Models [11] (Fig. 16.2)

Concept—This uses software which is used in CT scans to replicate various anatomic variations of the kidney and pelvicalyceal system. 3D printing of the models is done using water-soluble plastic embedded in silicone. The casts are dissolved, and it leaves a silicone model with a cavity inside to replicate the kidney. Sheets of foam replicate the skin and deeper muscles between the skin punctate point and kidney model.

Park et al. have evaluated a model to replicate the natural anatomy and variations of the pelvicalyceal system of the kidney. The authors claim that a range of models reflecting the variety and complexity of anatomy are available. It accurately replicates the anatomic architecture and orientation of the human renal collecting system.

The drawback of these systems is the need to use fluoroscopy and hence radiation and its side effects. A limitation of the model is its inability to use ultrasonography. The other disadvantage is poor haptics due to the silicon used. These models are expensive due to the need to use CT scan, 3D printing, and casting of each model individually.

16.4.4 Rawandale's PCNL Simulator [12] (Fig. 16.3)

Concept—This uses fluoroscopy with low settings of 50 kV and 0.6 mA. This has been designed using Computer Assisted Designing software (CAD). The models use acrylic, wood, and simple electronics. This is a low-cost model using locally available materials.

A cassette made up of polyvinyl foams of variable density, plastic films and aluminium foils simulates the parietal wall and retroperitoneum. When placed on the operating table, the model simulates a patient torso. A designed radio-opaque silicon kidney with a radiolucent pelvicalyceal system (PCS) serves as a puncturing target and replicates the model of an air pyelogram. Any access technique can be used with the model. A successful puncture is confirmed by returning fluid which can be pushed through the ureter of the silicon kidney. The model has the option of using a 4 mm telescope/ureteroscope attached to an endoscope camera system which can be positioned in the pelvicalyceal system via the ureter. This helps to visually confirm the accuracy of a successful puncture. On successful puncture, a wire is then parked into the PCS and sequential tract dilation is performed. Placement of the access sheath allows nephroscopy and stone manipulation.

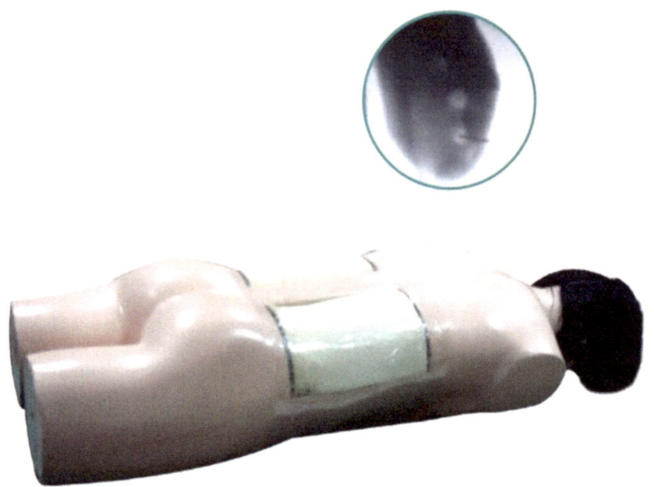

Fig. 16.3 Rawandale's fluoroscopy-based PCNL simulator

The spine, ribs and great vessels activate an electronic beep when the initial puncture needle (IPN) touches it. Alarms which indicate overshooting can also be incorporated. The major advantage is the respiratory kidney excursions replicated by a cam arrangement.

The authors claim this to be a mid-fidelity, low cost, fluoroscopy-compatible simulator which allows training in the OR environment providing near-natural tissue haptics. It aids in understanding the 3D renal and retroperitoneal anatomy and trains in the manipulation of fluoroscopy. Different kidney models can provide various operative scenarios of the kidney. It allows training with usual instruments, wires and catheters. It provides accurate feedback provided by simple electronics to ensure sufficient trainee guidance. It is portable and weighs 5.79 kg. The parietal wall cassette and the designed kidney allow for up to 300 punctures. This indirectly decreases the maintenance cost. The kidney cradle is also compatible with an animal kidney. A primary study has provided positive evidence for the simulator as a training and evaluation tool.

16.5 Biological Bench Models

Concept—Real tissue haptics cannot be replicated using synthetic material such as silicone or plastic. The porcine model provides a reasonable live surrogate for the human kidney. Hence some investigators have used live tissue in the simulators.

At least two groups of investigators have incorporated harvested porcine kidney/ureter units and mounted them to be viewed radiologically. Hammond et al. [13]

filled cadaver porcine kidney collecting systems with pebbles to simulate stones. They placed each renal/ureteral unit inside a chicken carcass. All tasks done by trainees such as fluoroscopic guided percutaneous renal puncture, guide wire placement, tract dilation, retrograde and antegrade pyelograms and rigid and flexible nephroscopy mimic real surgical steps giving structured training. No formal validation studies have been performed through a group of resident participants perceived that the model improved their comfort with the equipment and techniques of renal access and constituted a valuable experience.

Strohmaier and Giese [14] secured the renal units on a rectangular silicone mould. The entire assembly was covered with liquid silicone to embed the kidneys. The distal ureters remained accessible for retrograde contrast or fluid injection. Fluoroscopy and ultrasound-guided, percutaneous needle puncture and guide wire passage are performed. Tract dilation, sheath placement and nephroscopy can be performed. The model has good tissue haptics.

16.5.1 Vegetable Model

Concept—Use of easily available organic material such as vegetables to simulate puncture scenarios. Obviously, these are easy-to-obtain, cost-effective models.

Sinha and Krishnamoorthy [15] have published the use of an easily replicable vegetable simulator. It orients the trainees to depth and distance perception in PCNL scenarios. This model uses contrast-impregnated cotton balls. These serve as targets. These are embedded at staggered levels into one side of the bottle gourd. Trainees were made to target these using puncture needles. Satisfactory feedback was obtained by the examiners in this study (Fig. 16.4a, b).

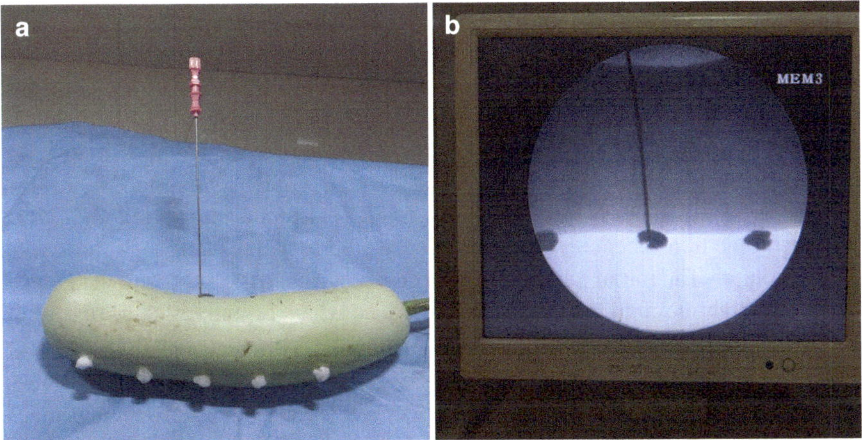

Fig. 16.4 Vegetable model. (**a**) Needle positioning using vegetable model. (**b**) C-arm image showing accuracy of needle puncture

16.6 Low-Fidelity Fluoroscopy Free Simulators

16.6.1 SimPortal CAT Simulation Model

Concept—This uses a mini C-arm and a silicon flank simulation model [19]. Includes a mini C-arm for simulating fluoroscopic imaging and a silicon flank simulation model. The C-arm has two mounted video cameras and is joined to tilt. These cameras produce a picture onto a monitor to simulate fluoroscopy image. The flank model has an anatomical cast of the upper urinary tract with an overlay of ribs. This tactically simulates the 10th–12th ribs. The simulated image is viewed on a computer screen for real-time visualization. The advantage of the model is the low cost and avoiding the side effects of radiation.

This is an attractive concept and relatively cheaper than VR simulators. The SimPortal haptics are difficult and hard. It is impossible to puncture the silicon slab with bare fingers on the initial puncture needle. The needle is provided with an extra-large hub to counter this problem. Multiple punctures render the whole silicon block void of clear vision. This needs replacement and may not be as cheap. The difficulties of this model also include dilatation and stone manipulation.

16.6.2 Rawandale's Virtual Fluoroscopy PCNL Simulator (Fig. 16.5 a, b)

Concept—Mid-fidelity segment simulator without fluoroscopy. The authors have designed a portable virtual fluoroscopy PCNL simulator. It was patented by the authors. It uses shadows against the light principle to produce a satisfactory resemblance of the virtual fluoroscopy image. It was designed using Computer Assisted Designing software (CAD). It is constructed using acrylic sheets, aluminium components, a point light source and a translucent interface.

This simulator uses an isocentric C-arm. The lower-end X-ray tube is replaced with a 12-V light source emitting visible light. The X-ray camera at the upper end is replaced with a high-definition camera. The C-arm is fixed so that the camera views the lamp through a translucent interface. The acrylic mannequin simulates a human torso. A metallic kidney pelvicalyceal system replica is suspended below the translucent screen at the point of isocentricity. This produces a black-and-white shadow on the translucent screen which is captured by the camera and reproduced on the monitor. The initial puncture (IP) needle is advanced to approach the kidney against the light through the translucent interface which resembles skin. An on/off foot switch operates the lamp and the camera. This produces a fluoroscopy-like picture on the monitor on pressing the footswitch. During the procedure, the trainee turns the "C" arm and attempts to visualize the kidney from a different angle. This step is the same as done during the actual surgery. The image quality may be fine-tuned on the monitor just like the conventional X-ray machine. The metallic pelvicalyceal system activates an electronic beep when touched with the initial puncture needle (IPN). This indicates the endpoint of the task. The mannequin has

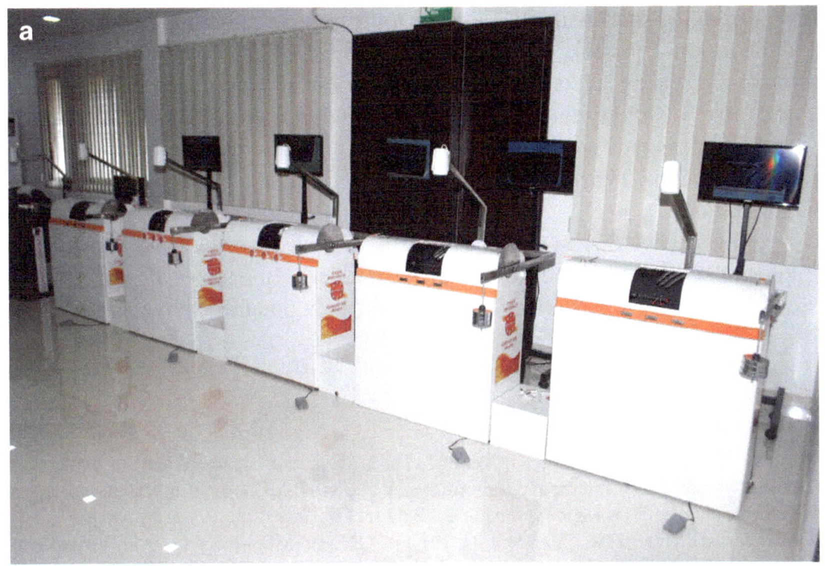

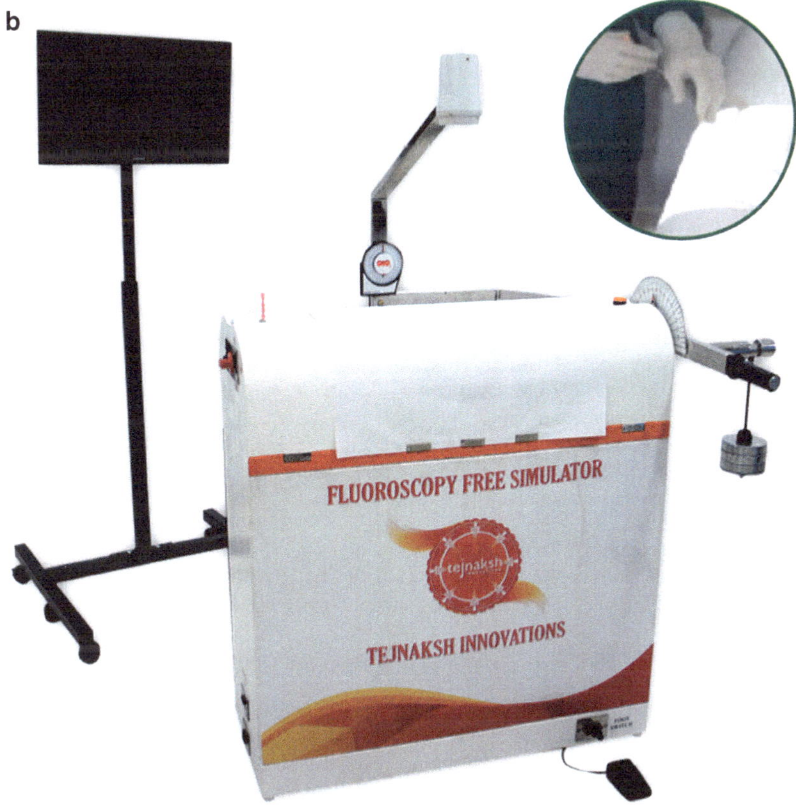

Fig. 16.5 (a, b) Rawandale's virtual fluoroscopy simulator

windows from the sides with HD cameras to inspect the puncture during and at the end of the task. Respiratory kidney excursions are replicated by a motorized CAM arrangement. Training levels are graded using various shapes of targets. A favourable face and content validity have been demonstrated in a phase 1 study done by the experts. These systems are low-cost as they do not employ computerized systems like the VR systems. They are cheap to produce and maintain. They do not have any radiation hazards.

The drawback of this system is the lack of objective feedback. There is no scoring, unlike sophisticated computerized models. But these allow trainees to replicate all steps of the PCNL procedure while being mentored by the trainer.

References

1. Michel MS, Knoll T, Kohrmann KU, Alken P. The URO mentor: development and evaluation of a new computer-based interactive training system for virtual life-like simulation of diagnostic and therapeutic endourological procedures. BJU Int. 2002;89:174.
2. Gallagher AG, Ritter EM, Champion H, Higgins G, Fried MP, Moses G, et al. Virtual reality simulation for the operating room: proficiency-based training as a paradigm shift in surgical skills training. Ann Surg. 2005;241:364.
3. Gallagher AG, Ritter EM, Satava RM. Fundamental principles of validation, and reliability: rigorous science for the assessment of surgical education and training. Surg Endosc. 2003;17:1525.
4. de la Rosette JJ, Laguna MP, Rassweiler JJ, Conort P. Training in percutaneous nephrolithotomy—a critical review. Eur Urol. 2008;54:994–1001.
5. Allen D, et al. Defining the learning curve for percutaneous nephrolithotomy. J Endourol. 2005;19:279–82.
6. Tanriverdi O, et al. The learning curve in the training of percutaneous nephrolithotomy. Eur Urol. 2007;52:206–12.
7. Kim SC, Kuo RL, Lingeman JE. Percutaneous nephrolithotomy: an update. Curr Opin Urol. 2003;13:235.
8. Astroza G, et al. Effect of supine vs prone position on outcomes of percutaneous nephrolithotomy in staghorn calculi: results from the Clinical Research Office of the Endourology Society Study. Urology. 2013;82:1240–5.
9. Kopta JA. The development of motor skills in orthopedic education. Clin Orthop. 1971;75:80.
10. Fitts PM, Posner MI. Human performance. Belmont: Brooks/Cole; 1967.
11. Park S, Matsumoto ED, Knudsen BE, et al. Face, content and construct validity testing on a percutaneous renal access simulator [abstract].
12. Rawandale ref fluoro.
13. Hammond L, Ketchum J, Schwartz BF. A new approach to urology training: a laboratory model for percutaneous nephrolithotomy. J Urol. 2004;172:1950–2.
14. Strohmaier WL, Giese A. Ex vivo training model for percutaneous renal surgery. Urol Res. 2005;33:191–3.
15. Sinha M, Krishnamoorthy V. Use of a vegetable model as a training tool for PCNL puncture. Indian J Urol. 2015;31:156–9.
16. Mahadevappa M. Patient radiation exposure issues. Radiographics. 2001;21:1033–45.
17. Knudsen BE, Matsumoto ED, Chew BH, et al. A randomized, controlled, prospective study validating the acquisition of percutaneous renal collecting system access skills using a computer based hybrid virtual reality surgical simulator: phase I. J Urol. 2006;176(5):2173–8.

18. Margulis V, Matsumoto ED, Knudsen BE, Chew BH, Pautler SE, Cadeddu JA, Denstedt JD, Pearle MS. Percutaneous renal collecting system access: can virtual reality shorten the learning curve? J Urol. 2005;173(suppl):315.
19. Veneziano D, Smith A, Reihsen T, Speich J, Sweet RM. The SimPORTAL fluoro-less C-arm trainer: an innovative device for percutaneous kidney access. J Endourol. 2015;29(2):240–5.
20. Adams F, Qiu T, Mark A, et al. Soft 3D-printed phantom of the human kidney with collecting system. Ann Biomed Eng. 2017;45:963–72. https://doi.org/10.1007/s10439-016-1757-5.

Tips and Tricks for PCNL

17

Sanjay Deshpande and Subodh R. Shivde

17.1 Preoperative Imaging

1. Study the IVP well—what to look for?
   (a) Relation of the stone to the PCS and ureter
   (b) Size of the stone—single or multiple
   (c) Preferably prone film
   (d) Size and site of the calyces
   (e) Size of the infundibula- Narrow means difficult to puncture if not impossible
   (f) Stone in calyceal diverticulum
   (g) Malrotated kidney—horse-shoe kidney
   (h) Size of the ureter
   (i) Decide which calyx to puncture
2. In a patient with Cironic Renal Failure and patient with radiolucent stones you have to rely on USG and CT scan findings hence study them well.
3. Dilute the contrast significantly approximately 20 mL of Urografin with 50 mL of N/S. Injection to be done slowly by the assistant otherwise PCS becomes too dark and obscures stones as well.
4. Watch the monitor continuously while injecting the contrast to study relation of the PCS to the stone.
5. When PCS is filled inject 5–10 mL of air. Often posterior calyces show up as white blobs in contrast to dark dyed filled anterior calyces. Quite often these are more medial than anterior calyces.
6. Remember the rule

S. Deshpande
Solapur, Maharashtra, India

S. R. Shivde (✉)
Department of Urology, Deenanath Mangeshkar Hospital and Research Centre, Pune, Maharashtra, India

S. R. Shivde (ed.), *Techniques in Percutaneous Renal Stone Surgery*, https://doi.org/10.1007/978-981-19-9418-0_17

Brodel 70% Posterior calyces are lateral and 30% anterior calyces are medial. This applies to the right kidney.

Hodgson 70% Posterior calyces are medial and 30% posterior calyces are lateral. This applies to the left kidney.

17.2 Study the Patient's Parameters

17.2.1 Per-operative Considerations

CBC, creatinine, BSL, BT, PT, platelets, blood group, HBs Ag, HIV, Blood Pressure, ECG, 2D echo, IVP study or USG or CT scan. Keep one unit of Blood ready.

If patient has a staghorn calculus, inform the patient that he/she may need 2–3 punctures or 2 sittings. It is possible that complete clearance may not be achieved.

17.2.2 Points to Consider in the Operative Room

Give good dose of broad-spectrum antibiotic with adequate cover for Gram negative organisms.

When turning prone take care of ET tubes, use eye pads for corneal protection. After turning first take both shoulders and hands out gradually and gently rotating shoulder and elbow joints. Then pay attention to pressure points like knees, ankles, if available use silicone pads. Use extra trolley with pillows to protect ankles and feet.

Protect ureteric catheter. It may get pulled down accidentally. Some surgeons keep guidewire in situ until the final position of ureteric catheter in prone position is seen. This may facilitate re-insertion of ureteric catheter in case of accidental displacement.

Connect Foleys catheter to urosac bag, which is hung on the same side as surgeon so that color of the urine can be seen.

If patient is diabetic, monitor BSL intraoperatively as hypoglycemia may cause undesirable physiological consequences.

17.2.3 Surgical Trouble Shooting

17.2.3.1 Access Difficulty

A. **Unable to pass a guidewire or ureteric catheter**

   This may happen due to edema of the ureteric orifice or prolonged use of stent and may sometimes lead to submucosal passage of guidewire leading to a false passage. A blood-stained discharge from the ureteric opening is the hint to it and from here one needs to proceed with caution. The use of a small caliber ureteroscope either 4 Fr or 6 Fr is strongly advised at this stage as it will allow the operator to enter the lumen of the ureter leading to a safe passage of guidewire up to the pelvicalyceal system.

B. Difficulty during the passage of guidewire into the system

1. Ureteric catheter does not go into the PCS due to stone impacted at PUJ. **Solution:**
   - Keep the catheter at PUJ and change to zebra guidewire if you have used Terumo type flexible tip wire first. A small caution about use of zebra wire is that sharp end may cause perforation of the system and false passages.
   - Flush with normal saline to create some space between the stone and the wall of the ureter, to displace the stone. An attempt is made to pass the guidewire. If this is not feasible, then keep the tip of ureteric catheter just below the PUJ and inject diluted contrast to see if it gets into PCS fine. The next step is to make the patient prone and do the routine initial puncture.
   - If contrast medium does not go into PCS, then do blind puncture using Chiba or lumbar puncture needle at the junction of 12th rib and lateral border of erector spinae which is the usual site of renal pelvis. This is *blind puncture technique*. If you get urine, then inject diluted contrast to opacify the PCS system and then proceed with IP.
   - Other alternatives are
     - Give IV contrast and wait for contrast to fill the PCS like IVP
     - OR do PCN under *USG guidance.*
2. In left PCNL, keep the calyx to be punctured at 10 clock position on the monitor. In right PCNL, keep the calyx to be punctured at 11 o'clock on the monitor. These positions will give maximum distance visibility of the needle tip from start till PCS entry.
3. Adjust *direction of the needle when "C" ARM is at 0°* under the following criteria:
   (a) Axis—posterior to anterior, lateral to medial
   (b) Target—tip of the calyx to be punctured (fornix)
   (c) Direction should be toward the center of the calyx
   (d) Direction should be toward the center of the renal pelvis
   (e) Do not cross puncture infundibulum
4. How to decide which calyx to be punctured?
   (a) The calyx through which maximum stone bulk can be cleared
   (b) Calyx should be in straight alignment to the axis of puncture

Please refer to Fig. 17.1 showing the target trajectory to a large pelvic stone by planning to hit the middle calyx but this would miss a significant lower calyx stone chunk so the point of entry changed to the lower calyx making the stones accessible in one puncture (Fig. 17.2). Also note the significant dilatation of calyx making the puncture relatively easy.

5. When to go for upper calyceal puncture?
   (a) When maximum stone bulk is in upper calyx or infundibulum with dilated upper calyx
   (b) When upper calyx cannot be reached through lower calyx
   (c) Stone at PUJ or upper ureter—when axis is straight to approach PUJ or upper ureter

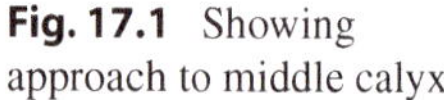
Fig. 17.1 Showing approach to middle calyx

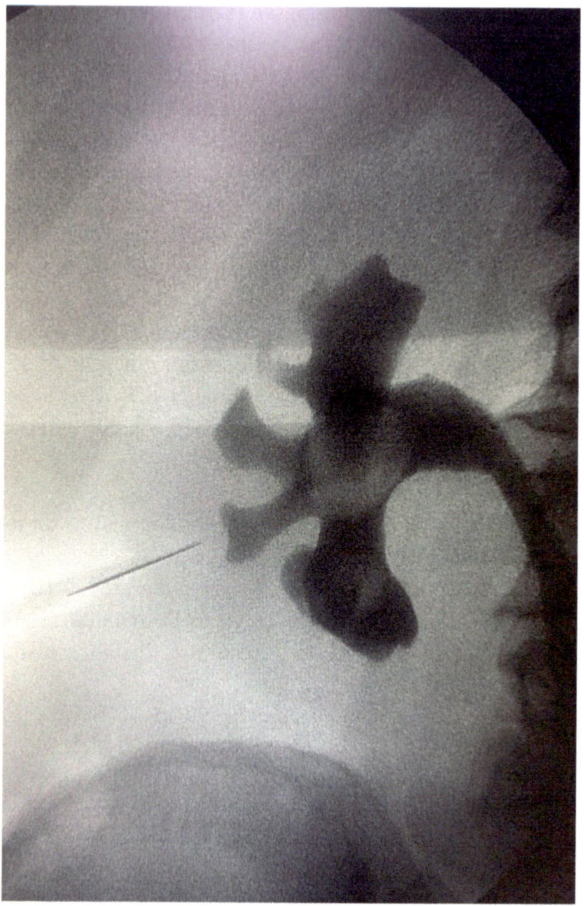

6. Stand close to OT table and patient for lower calyceal puncture. Position monitor of "C" ARM either at head end next to anesthetist for lower calyceal puncture or at lower side or near control panel close to the X-ray technician for upper calyceal puncture
7. Adjust for middle calyceal puncture cephalic caudal lateral medial on the monitor in relation to prone position of the patient before anesthesia is given
   - Use ALARA principle to reduce radiation. Tie back of the lead apron with bandage to prevent it from sliding on to your shoulder to reduce your shoulder pain
   - Use head end controlled radiolucent OT table. If not available have radiolucent extensions at the lower end or have complete wooden table
   - Adjust (reduce or increase) brightness on the monitor to eliminate peripheral whiteness so that only PCS is seen
   - Think before or after exposure and not when II shoot is on
   - If possible, have foot control for "C" ARM
   - Adjust KV and MAS as per the patient's requirements

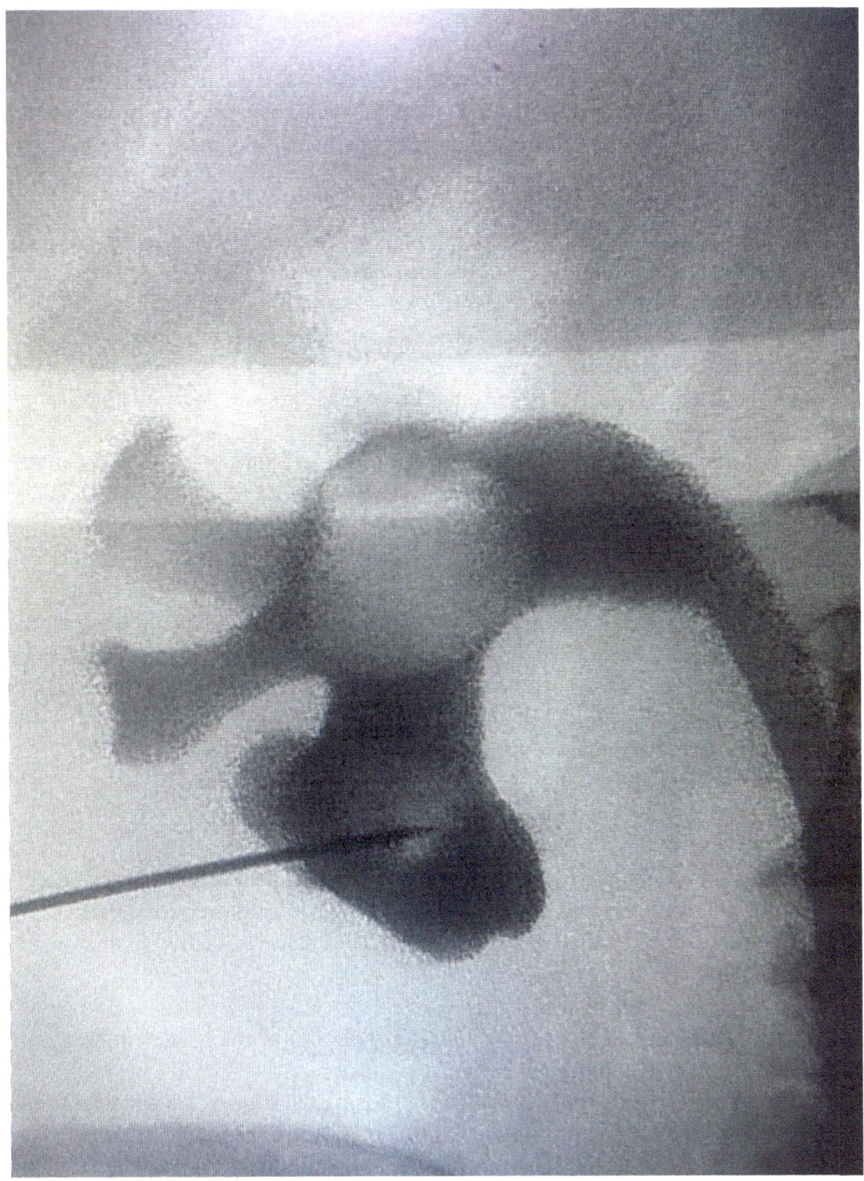

Fig. 17.2 Showing lower calyx approach to target both the stones

8. How do you know that you are near the calyx?

   Kidney moves (medially) when the needle touches the capsule of the kidney. This manoeuvre is called "jiggling". Then you know that you are close to the region. On puncturing the desired calyx you see the ''Fovea Sign''with the indentation of cup of calyx.

   Then go in further when you feel a "give way" which indicates that mostly you have entered the calyx.

Then remove the stillette and aspirate with 2 cc syringe, a clear return of urine indicates correct puncture.

Point of value is to send the aspirated fluid for culture and sensitivity tests as any post-operative fever or septicemia may have to be treated aggressively and a spectrum of antibiotics would then allow the team to control sepsis based on these reports [1].

9. What if you get blood?

   Either you are in opposite cortex (zone beyond the calyx) or in the proximal cortex meaning you have not yet reached the desired calyx.

   Solution: Withdraw the needle and keep aspirating.

   If you get clear fluid well and good—it means that you have come into the calyx. If no fluid comes despite continuous withdrawal and only blood comes it means you were short. Check on IITV. Come out. Flush the needle with normal saline.

   PLEASE REPEAT THE STEP!
10. Further attempt-same thing keeping needle in place turn the "C" ARM to 30° and assess the depth [2]. Please refer to the Sect. 2.6, 2.7 and 2.8 in Chapter 2.
11. If blood-stained fluid is aspirated not just blood, then try flushing with N/S from below to see if this clears.
12. What is 2-part and 3-part needle?

    2 part is needle sheath with stillette. The tip of stillette should be diamond shaped and not beveled. The tip of needle sheath should be flat and atraumatic and not beveled. Eco tip needle is used in USG guided punctures as the eco tip increases the echogenicity—helping the puncture (Fig. 17.3).

    3-part needle has outer shaft with flat atraumatic tip
    - Inner shaft with beveled tip
    - Stillette with beveled tip

The outer shaft is supposed to be of larger diameter and shorter and inner shaft is longer thinner—18 G. So that less traumatic (Fig. 17.4). If confirmed in the system, then outer shaft can be pushed down and inner one is removed. Through this second safety guidewire can also be placed.

13. Guidewire does not enter the PCS and tip goes out of the system although on aspiration fluid is coming out

    Don't be satisfied—mostly needle is touching the edge of the calyceal lining with cortical tissue. Withdraw a few millimeters and change the direction of the needle. Insert the needle further—the guidewire must fold as per the contours of PCS (Fig. 17.5) if not withdraw the needle and make a fresh puncture.
14. When you choose a calyx:
    (a) see its relation to the 12th rib
    (b) see the infundibulum

    As much as possible—try and negotiate to pass the guidewire into the ureter by simple angulation of the needle tip towards the pelviureteric junction, if not possible at least into the upper calyx (Fig. 17.5).

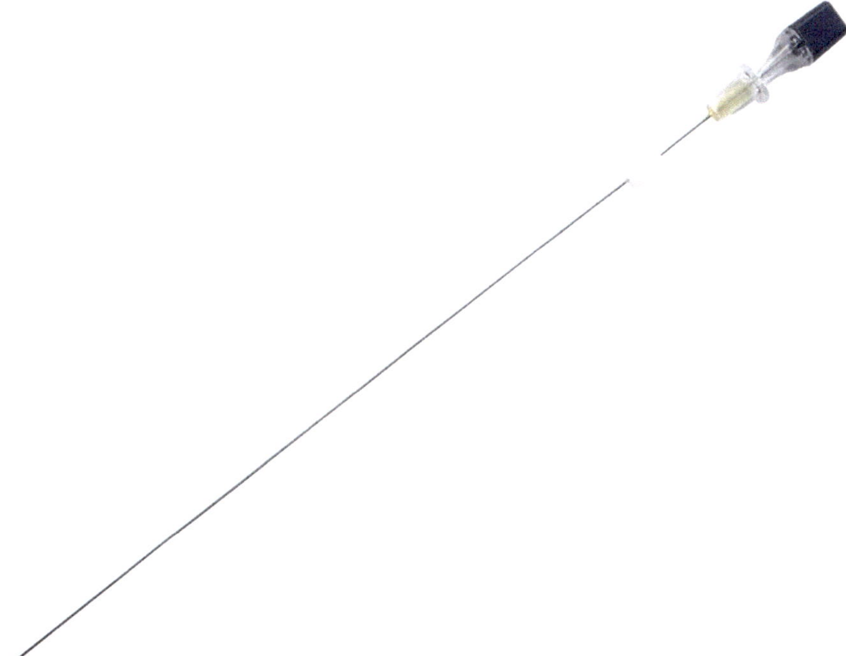

Fig. 17.3 2-part needle

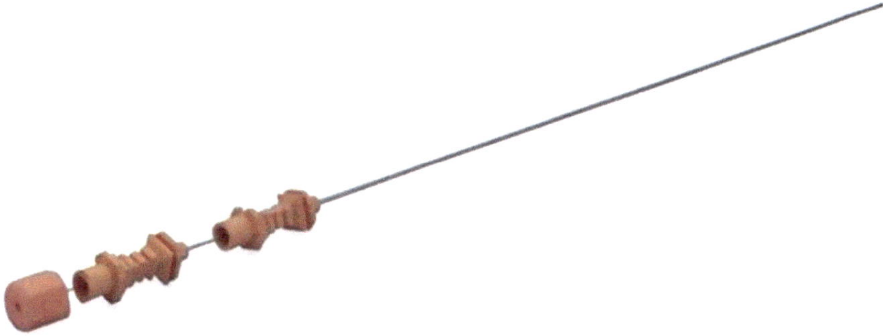

Fig. 17.4 3-part needle

15. Guidewire—PTFE—J tipped
    - Terumo straight or J tipped
    - Mixture of flexible + stiff wire

We strongly recommend the use of 2 wires to ensure the completion of a procedure without the loss of access (Fig. 17.6).

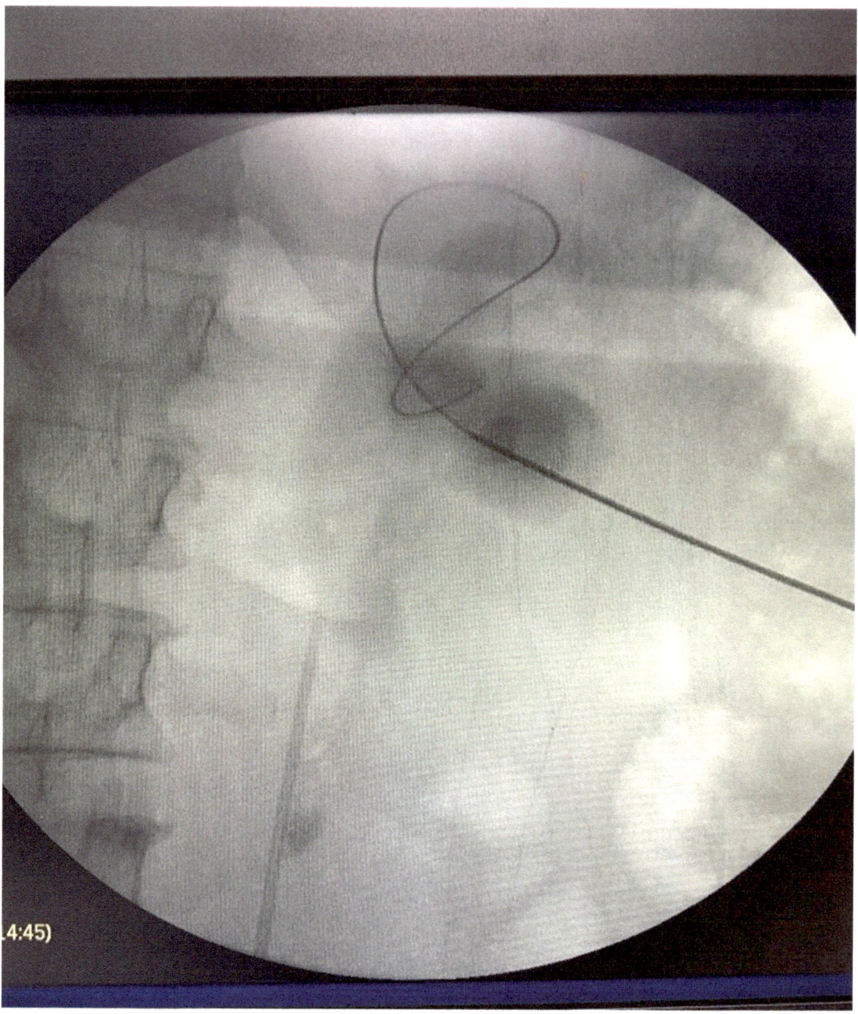

Fig. 17.5 Guidewire taking the contour of PCS

16. Incise liberally along the needle deep to divide the thoracolumbar fascia which is the first site of resistance during dilation.
17. In the upper calyceal puncture, ask the anesthetist to *hold the breath preferably in expiration*, approach intercostally from lateral to medial side *to avoid injury to the pleura* [3].
    - After obtaining fluid and passing guidewire, the direction of the needle can be changed to make it more vertical in alignment with the axis of the upper calyx and dilation can be carried out in this axis. This will reduce the torque and hence bleeding.

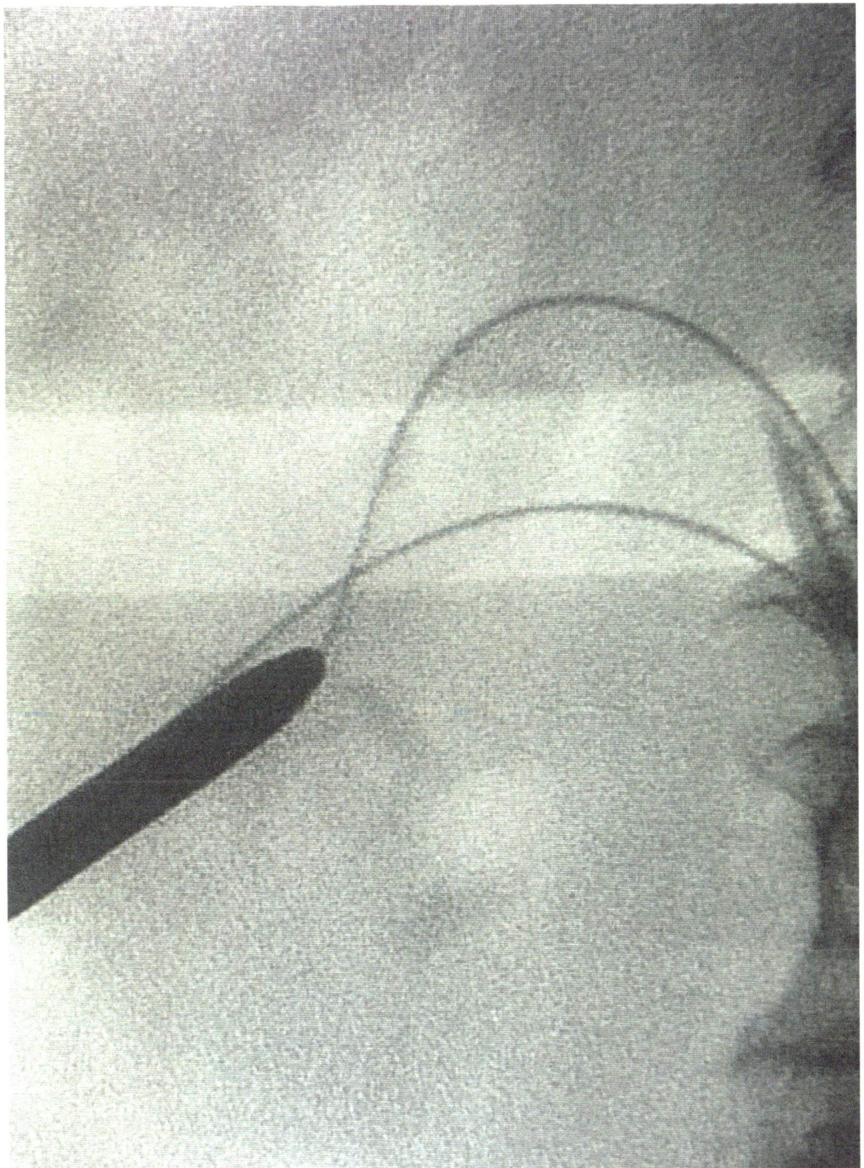

Fig. 17.6 Showing primary and safety wires in place during the dilation

18. After doing PCNL through the upper calyx, at the end check costophrenic angle on IITV to check for fluid collection or pneumothorax. If in doubt get chest X-ray done in the recovery room. If still in doubt portable USG of the chest is done to check for fluid or pneumothorax. Lastly plain CT-thorax can be done if still in doubt about the injury to pleura.

19. Initially use the screw dilator or serial facial dilators or Alken dilator cannula. While doing this buckling of the guidewire over the dilator can happen (Fig. 17.7). This happens at two places.
    (a) Thoracolumbar fascia
    (b) Renal capsule

As kidney moves with respiration the guidewire also moves. If it is PTFE, it bends and cannot be straightened.

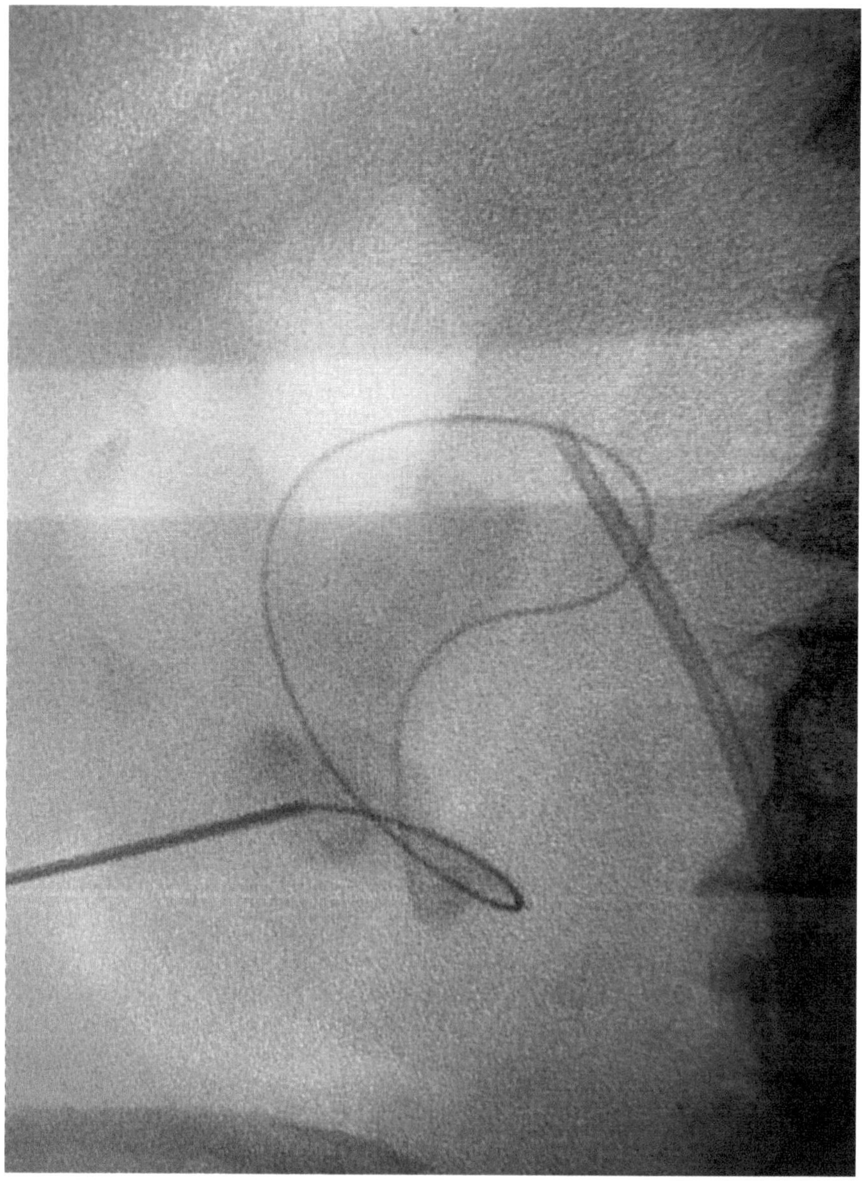

Fig. 17.7 Shows buckling of the guidewire

Solution:

A. Dilate in the same respiratory phase that you had done initial puncture.
B. To check angle turn "C" ARM to 30°, this will help to reduce buckling.
C. Withdraw the guidewire into the initial dilator and pass another guidewire. Or withdraw guidewire into the guide rod or Alken needle (Fig. 17.8).

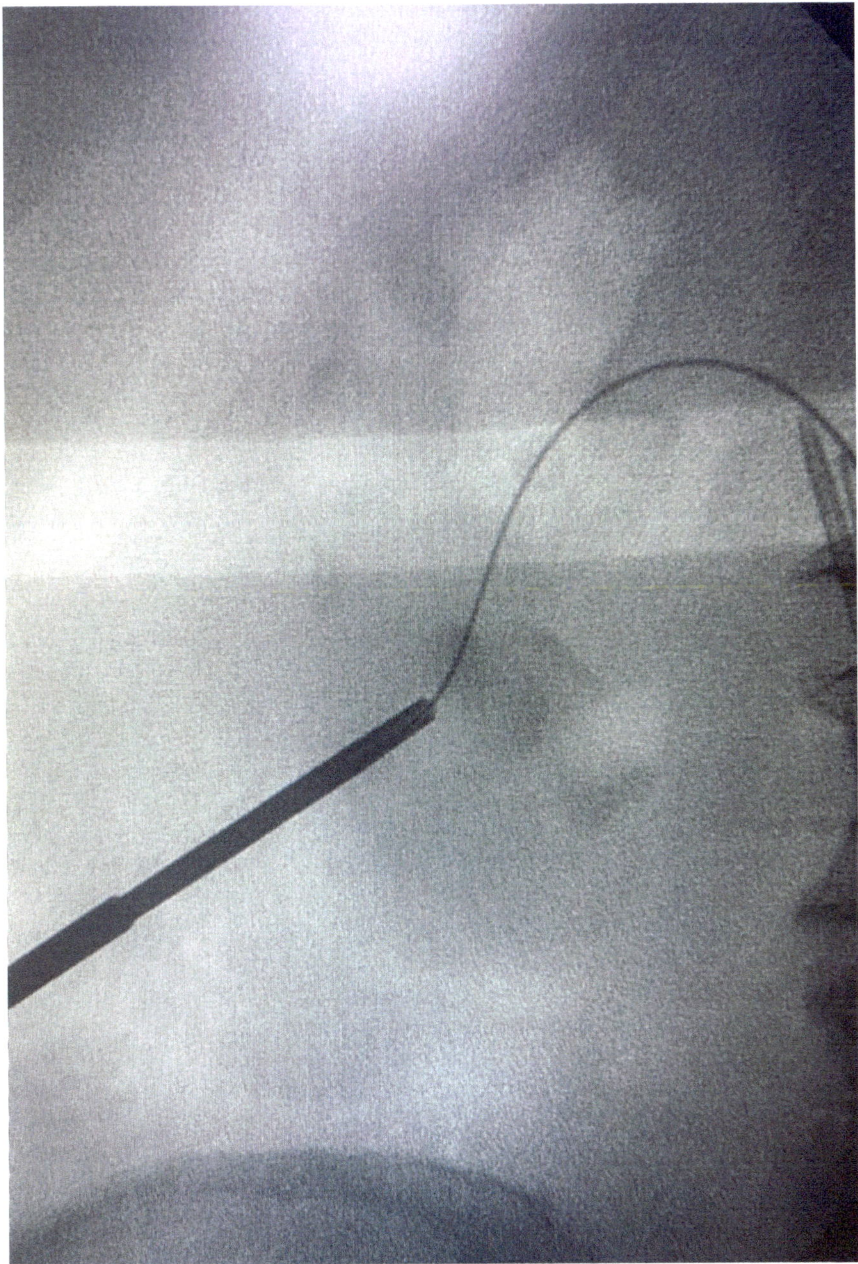

Fig. 17.8 Alken needle and sheath being used over the guidewire

20. Friction test: During every dilation guidewire should freely and smoothly move in the dilators if not, i.e. if there is friction it means that the angle of the dilator is not right so realign the dilator.
21. In previously operated patients, it may be tough to go through. Never put guide rod without initial dilation. If they do not pass, the reverse side of the guide rod can be used for initial dilatation and then the usual side.
22. Dilate up to the calyx under II TV. Beyond the calyx further dilation is done under vision using nephroscope unless the PCS is significantly dilated.
23. While dilating
    (a) Keep flushing from below through the ureteric catheter.
    (b) Put some contrast from below to know the edge of the calyx to know the limit of dilatation. Check within 0° and 30° of "C" ARM.
24. Dilators—Fascial Amplatz—Alken type with Alken rod and serial telescopic metal dilators. Balloon dilators with pressure gauge system.
25. If stone is occupying the calyx of puncture initially inject N/S through ureteric catheter to create space between stone and wall of the calyx before putting contrast. Then only you will get fluid on aspiration during initial puncture (IP). Guidewire may or may not go by the side of the stone, then curl it in the space only (Fig. 17.9).

In such a case dilate up to the stone only and not beyond, as invariably it goes through the cortical tissues and causes significant bleeding (Fig. 17.10). Stone clearance should be managed subsequently by Miniscope or conventional nephroscope to achieve a "stone free" status (Fig. 17.11).

26. During dilation:
    (a) Do not let guide rod go forward false as it may lead to perforation of pelvicalyceal system and false passages.
    (b) Keep guidewire in place.
    (c) Two sites of resistance are encountered during dilation they are at the level of (1) thoracolumbar fascia and (2) at the level of renal capsule.
        Hence with gentle thrust negotiate these areas.
27. During dilation the torso of the hand should be on the patient's hip and using wrist movements—dilator should be inserted using both screw (rotational) movement and gentle thrust.
    - The surgeon should always be in control of the dilator along with the guide rod and guidewire.
    - Some surgeons use both hands to insert dilators. Insert appropriate size snugly fitting with beveled edge Amplatz sheath.
28. When dilatation is done, we may use a purpose designed adhesive plastic drape (Fig. 17.12) with a collection channel attached to the tubing.

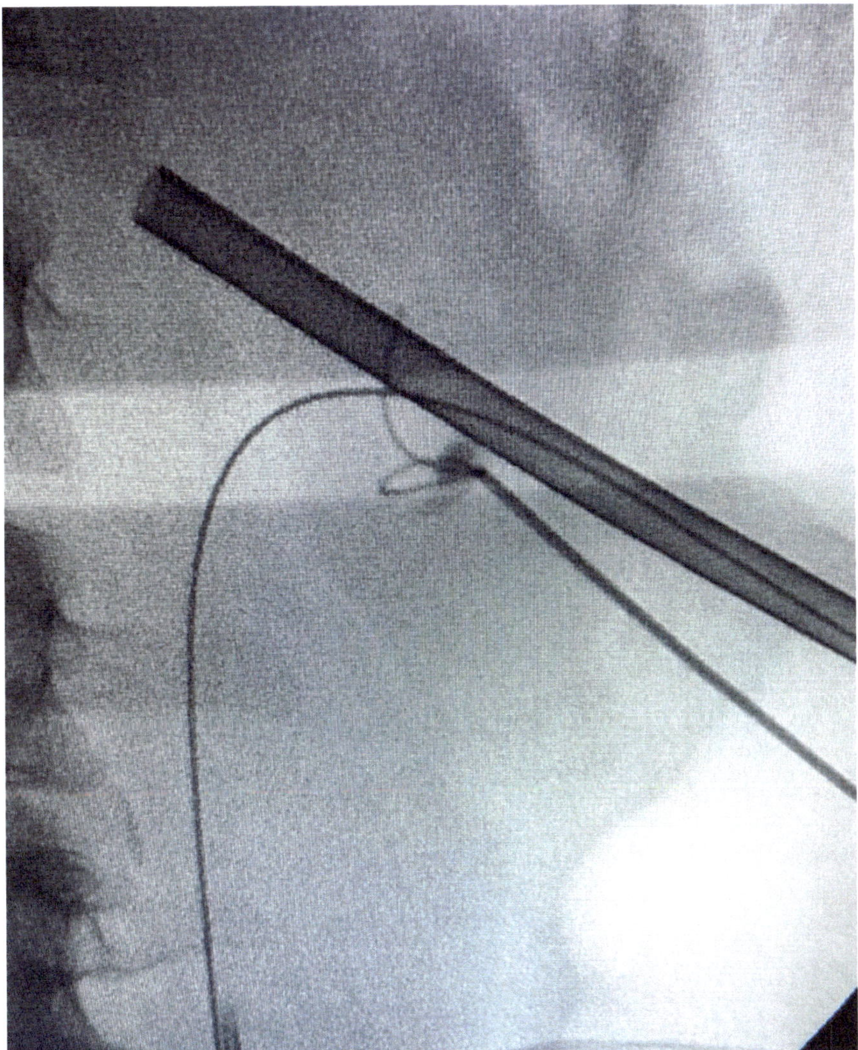

Fig. 17.9 Showing wire coiling in the calyx besides the stones and not entering the PCS

- Set 4 things—Nephroscope, camera and light source-cable, irrigation and lithotripsy device keep suction and flushing ready. Assemble everything. To flush use endotracheal suction tubes. Connect to 20 mL syringe and keep ready. Also keep endoscopic suction ready.
- We recommend keeping all these ready and then remove the dilators along with guide rod as waiting leads to tamponade.

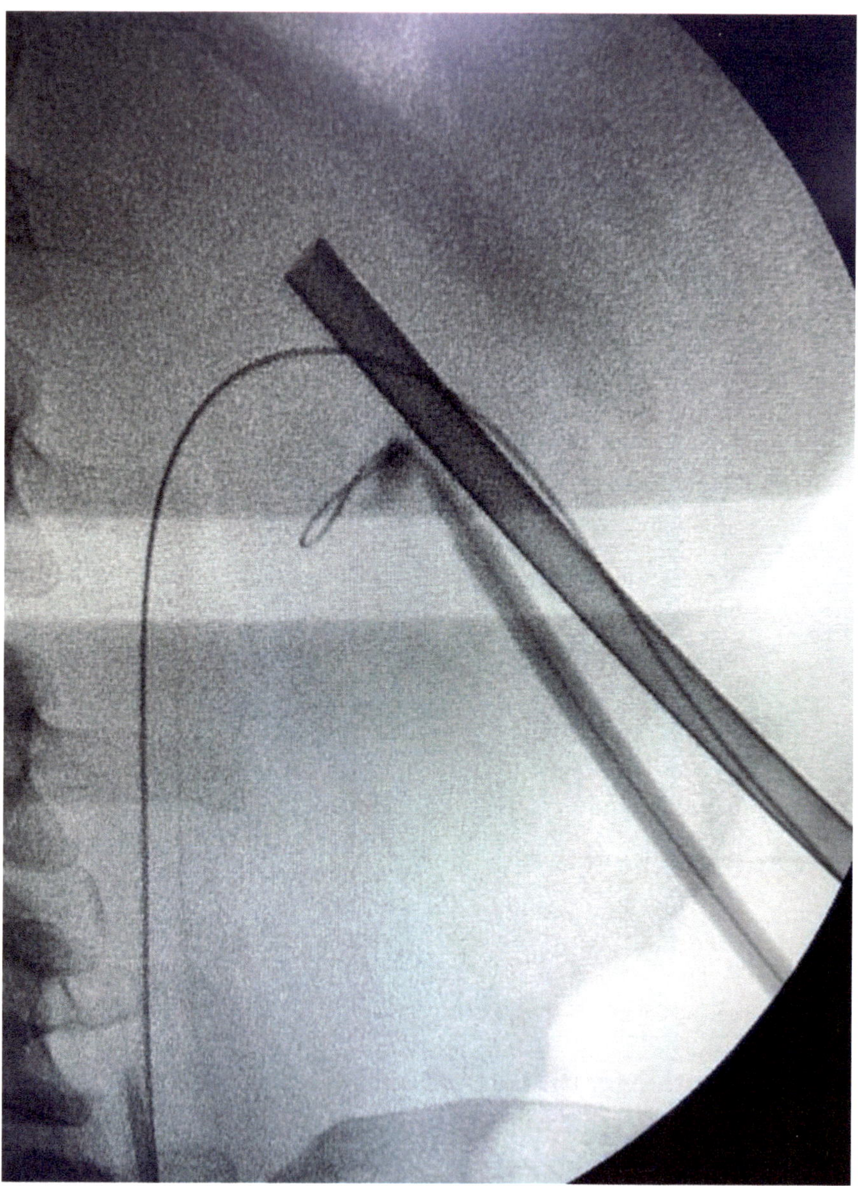

Fig. 17.10 Showing the screw dilator up to the stone over the coiled guidewire

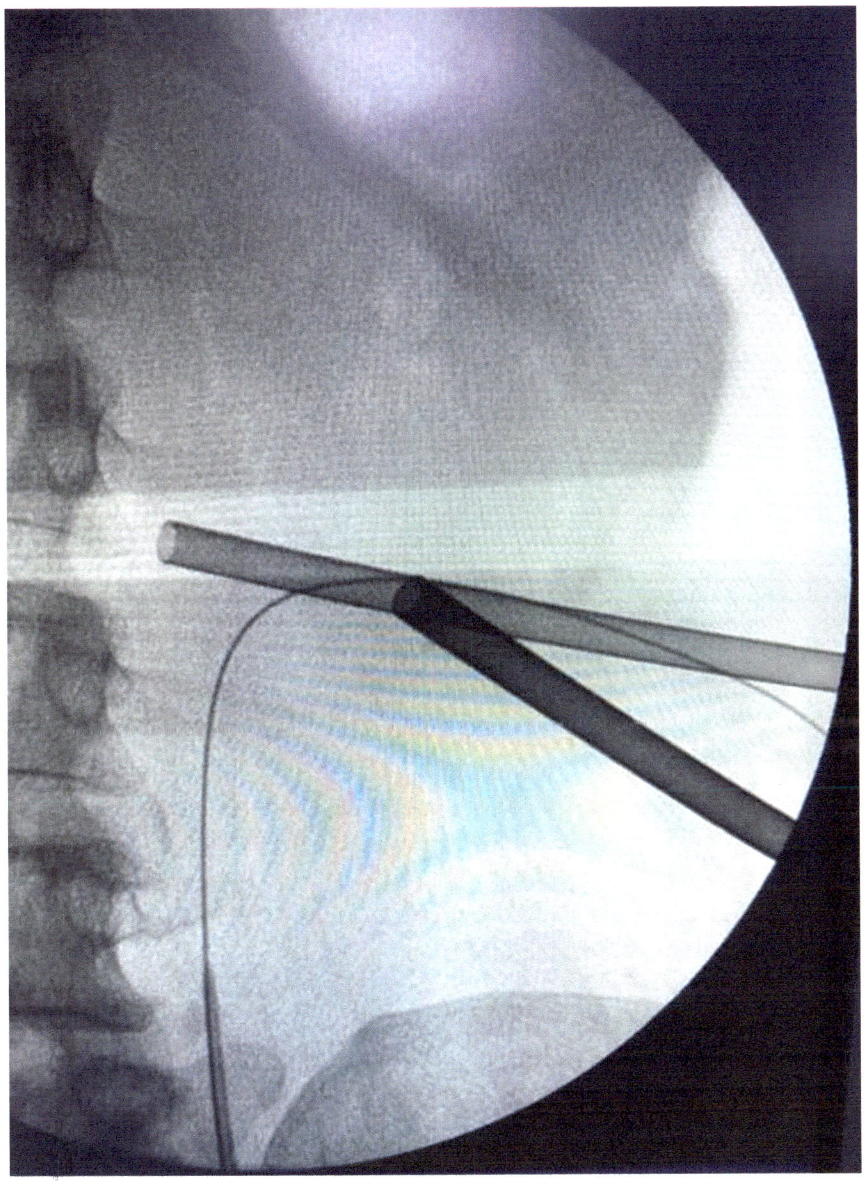

Fig. 17.11 Showing "stone free" status

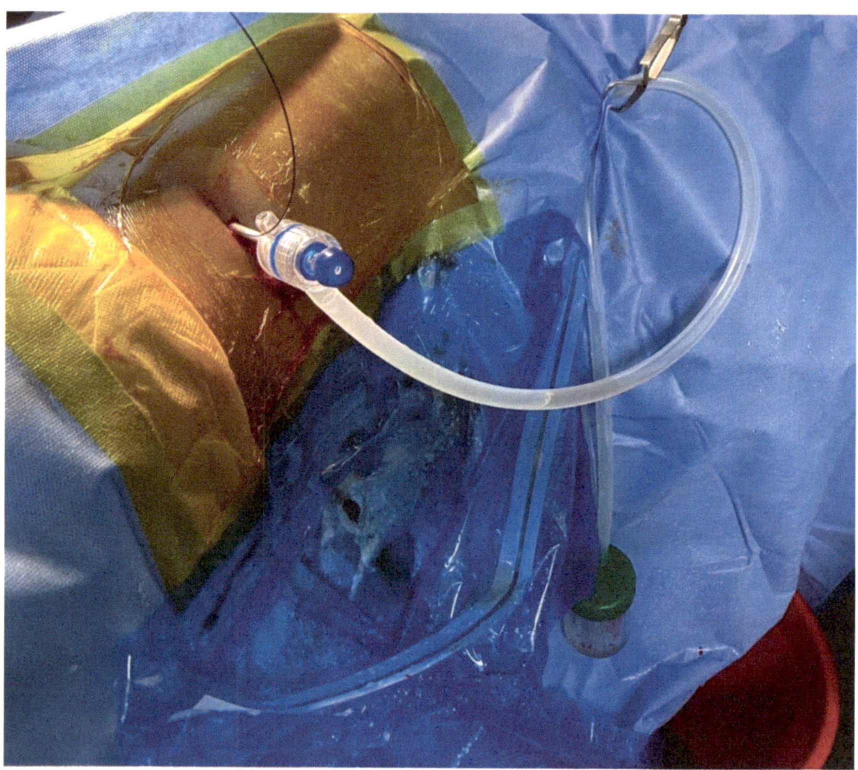

Fig. 17.12 Typical draping for PCNL with sheath in place with attached suction and cup for stone fragments

References

1. Webb DR. Routine PCNL. In: Percutaneous renal surgery. Cham: Springer; 2016. https://doi.org/10.1007/978-3-319-22828-0_5.
2. Rodrigues PL, Rodrigues NF, Fonseca J, Lima E, Vilaça JL. Kidney targeting and puncturing during percutaneous nephrolithotomy: recent advances and future perspectives. J Endourol. 2013;27(7):826–34.
3. Aro T, et al. V04-03 tips and tricks to avoid supracostal percutaneous nephrolithotomy access. J Urol. 2020;203(Suppl 4):e387–8.

Stone Evaluation—Biochemical Analysis and Its Clinical Implications

18

Sanjeev Mehta

18.1 Urinary Stone Evaluation in Laboratory: Why and How?

"Give me your stone and I will tell who you are!" [1].

The objective of stone analysis is to collect all the relevant information from the stone material helping the physician to establish causes of stone formation and growth.

This chapter highlights stone disease evaluation in the laboratory, its methods and usefulness in brief.

18.2 Why Do Stones Form?

18.2.1 Theories of Stone Formation in Brief

Supersaturation is believed to be the main force behind formation of stones. The other factors which are implicated are the physiological and metabolic factors. It was not until Pak et al. published an ambulatory protocol to test urine in 1975 that separation of various causes was possible [2]. The causes were differentiated as absorptive, resorptive and renal causes.

The other causes of stone formation are nucleation, aggregation and stone growth. The commonest type of stones are the calcium stones. We still do not have a very clear idea about all mechanisms of stone formation, and ongoing research allows us to evaluate the factors responsible and hence treatment options could evolve further. Idiopathic calcium stone formation has certain features, and they are: (1) variable urine values of all examined parameters, (2) stone formation is a form of concentration disorder and not just excretion of certain elements in excess [3].

S. Mehta (✉)
Uro Lab, Ahmedabad, India

S. R. Shivde (ed.), *Techniques in Percutaneous Renal Stone Surgery*, https://doi.org/10.1007/978-981-19-9418-0_18

It was not until Albright et al. published a case series of various biochemical abnormalities in a series of patients that some forms of calcium stone formation could be attributed to hypercalciuria without any cause. These patients showed increased calcium excretion, low phosphorus and normal serum calcium [4].

The other causes responsible for stone formation are an imbalance between the stone-promoting and stone-prevention factors. The known stone-prevention factors are magnesium, citrates and phosphorus. Some organic factors responsible for prevention are Tamm Horsfall protein, nephrocalcin. The factors known to promote stone formation are calcium, oxalate, urate, sodium, cystine, low urinary pH and bacterial products.

Renal stone analysis and 24 h urine metabolic tests with supersaturation index are special investigations requiring analytical expertise.

Kidney stones are classified into four major groups

1. Calcium stones (80%)
2. Uric acid stones (5–10%)
3. Struvite stones (10–15%)
4. Cystine stones (1–2%)

However, about 65 different chemical compounds are found in kidney stone, mostly in combination and sometimes in pure form also. Now with newer methods using latest technology, all these can be measured even if they are in very small percentage.

18.2.2 Algorithm for the Initial Evaluation of the Patient Presenting with a Kidney Stone

After obtaining a good history and family history of nephrolithiasis, a biochemical profile ordered would be serum sodium, potassium, chloride, bicarbonate, serum calcium, uric acid and phosphorus. A urine test for microscopy and culture would be ordered as well. And last but not the least a stone analysis.

A recurrent or metabolic stone former would be ordered to have a 24-h urine tests for biochemistry checking for volume and chemical composition of excreted urine. It would also involve measurement of supersaturation index.

1. Blood and urine tests
   (a) Blood tests—some significant observations
      Low potassium and bicarbonate indicate strong possibility of renal tubular acidosis.
      High uric acid indicates uric acid diathesis, uric acid stone.
      High calcium could imply primary hyperparathyroidism.
      Low phosphorus levels mean possible renal phosphorus leak.
      Parathyroid hormone elevated levels would prompt investigation for primary or secondary hyper parathyroid disorder.
   (b) Urine tests—significant findings
      pH more than7.5 suggests infective origin of stones.
      pH less than 6.5 suggests uric acid lithiasis.

Sediments with crystalluria.

Any indicators such as pyuria or bacterial presence in urine should hint towards urinary infection and triple phosphate stones.

2. Stone analysis:

A properly done stone analysis diagnoses metabolic abnormality, possible hint of infection stone and stone formation due to drugs.

18.3 Overview of Currently Used Techniques for Stone Analysis

1. Examination of available stone material is done and it is subjected to counting, noting sizes and external appearances. This is usually done before breaking down the stone. A visible nidus is hardly ever seen. A microscope may be used in case of smaller size of stones. A typical stone is seen as a crystalline form with radiating lattice pattern typical of each biochemical composition.
2. A small sized stone may not be suitable for above method of examination and thus a method called chromatography can be used. The principle used is difference in distribution patterns of a given chemical mixture.
3. Composition of stone when subjected to Fourier Infra-red Spectroscopy (FT-IR) or X-ray diffraction, i.e. exposure to monochromatic X-rays produces specific pattern. This may be called 'Fingerprints' of each type of stone. A computational software is used to identify the chemical composition.
4. Organic compounds such as stones when subjected to excitation by light of specific wavelength exabits fluorescence. This emits light of different wavelengths specific to chemical composition of the stone. This is suitable for a smaller amount of material.

   Other methods used for stone biochemical analysis are use of polarizing microscope, chemical microscopy and electron microscopy.

   Ultraviolet visible spectroscopy can be used for detection of stones made of drugs and drug metabolites.
5. Integrated crystallographic analysis (Fig. 18.1).
6. FT-IR (Fourier Transform Infrared Spectroscopy) (Fig. 18.2).

18.3.1 Composition and Hardness Factor of Stones and Its Significance

Here is the list of stones of varying hardness in the descending order. The hardness factor is given in bracket for each stone type.

Cystine (2.4), brushite (2.2), calcium oxalate monohydrate (com) (1.3), carbonate apatite (1.3), hydroxy apatite (1.1), calcium oxalate dihydrate (cod) (1), uric acid/urate (1), struvite (1), mixed stone (1).

The hardness factor or index indicates retreatment, increased number of ESWL sessions and higher index of energy required during treatments.

Patient's Name: xxx **Age/Sex:** **Date:**
Referred By : Dr. **Ref.No:**

INTEGRATED CRYSTALLOGRAPHIC ANALYSIS OF URINARY CALCULI

Gross and Micro-Chemical Analysis:

Specimen consists of multiple, irregular calculi totally weighing 3.43 gms and spreaded in area of 3.0 x 4.0 cms.The outer surface show white colored soft surface.

Calculi are composed of aggregates of fine orthorhombic crystals of magnesium ammonium phosphate hexahydrate, interspersed with deposits of microcrystalline and octahedral crystals of carbonate apatite. A protein matrix is demonstrated.

No distinct nidus is microscopically seen.

FT-IR Analysis: Fourier Transform Infrared Spectroscopy:

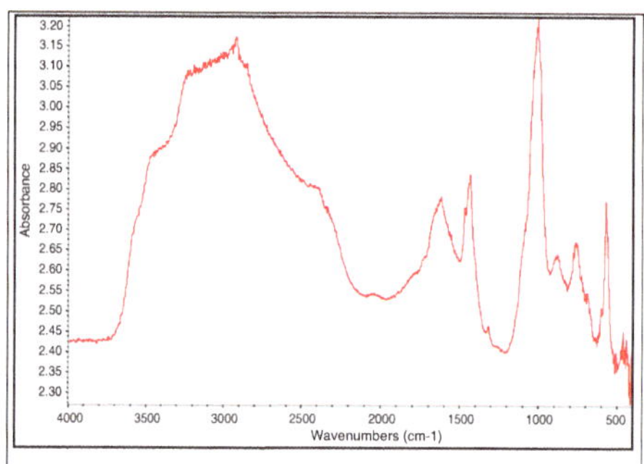

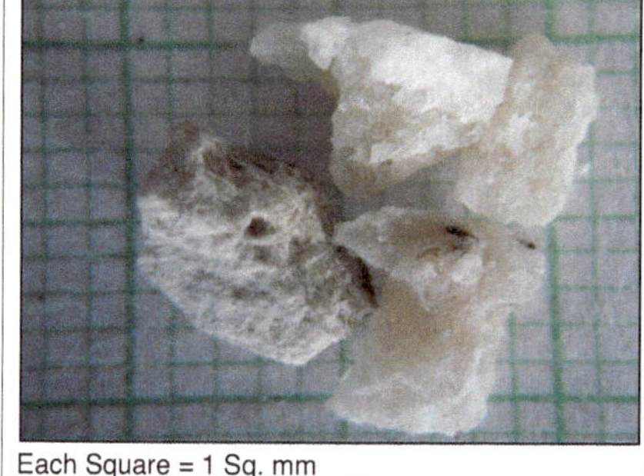

Each Square = 1 Sq. mm

*Photographs of all calculi not possible due to large photographs sizes.

Principal Stone Components (Results):

Chemical Name	Approximate Percentage	Mineralogical Name	Formula
Magnesium Ammonium Phosphate Hexahydrate	83 %	Struvite	$MgNH_4PO_4*6H_2O$
Dahllite	13 %	Carbonate Apatite	$Ca_{10}(PO_4)_2(CO_3)_6(OH)_2$
Protein and Blood	04 %		

DR.SANJEEV MEHTA
M.D.(Patho&Bio-Cryst.Analyst)

Fig. 18.1 Integrated crystallography analysis of stone

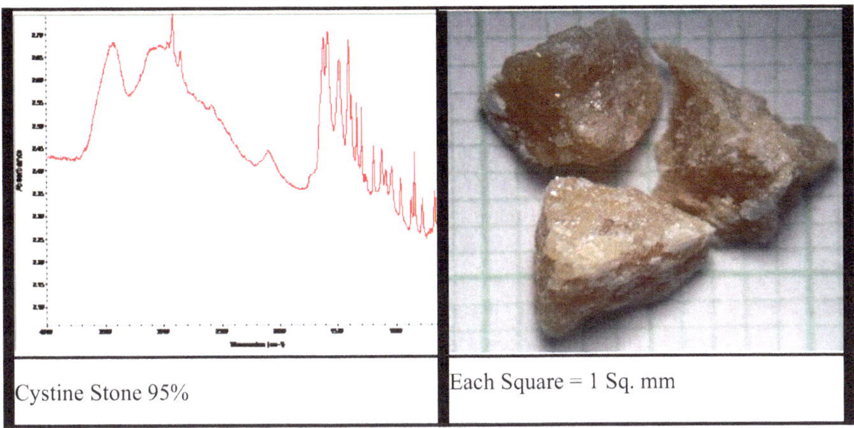

Fig. 18.2 FT-IR analysis of cysteine stone

18.3.2 Summary of Biochemical Abnormalities in Various Stone Compositions

1. Acidic urine with low urine volume and more excretion of oxalates is a feature of pure calcium stone formers. They exhibit higher serum calcium and hypercalciuria.
2. Calcium oxalate monohydrate stone formers show hypomagnesemia.
3. Calcium oxalate dihydrate stone formers show hypocitraturia.
4. Renal tubular acidosis is a feature carbonate apatite and brushite stones. These are often associated with hyperparathyroidism.
5. Struvite stones are infection stones of mixed composition (magnesium ammonium phosphate) having pH more than7.5. The commonest infective organism in such stones is proteus. Other organisms isolated in urine are *Pseudomonas*, *Staphylococcus*, *Klebsiella*, *E. coli*.
6. Ammonium urate stones are calcium containing stones and are associated with hyperuricosuria. In adults, they may be associated with recurrent infection.
7. Uric acid stones are having high uric acid in blood and urine. The patient may also be suffering from gout and of myeloproliferative disorder, the urinary pH in uric acid stone patient is 6.5 or less.
8. Cystine stones almost always occur in pure form and having cystinuria. Urine pH is highly acidic. Xanthene stones show xanthinuria. Both are autosomal recessive disorders and rare. Dihydroxyadenine and drug-induced stones like atazanavir, sulphadiazine can only be identified with the help newer methods of stone analysis.

18.3.3 What's New in Stone Composition Analysis?

Bargagli et al. published a series of patients with cardiovascular abnormalities with stone formation and a comparison group without stone formation tendency. They postulated that the underlying abnormality common to both groups, i.e. stone formers and cardiovascular diseases was the lower excretion of citrates and magnesium. Stone formers and arterial plaque formers have this common etiological factor. More prospective studies are needed to prove this hypothesis [5].

Artificial intelligence (AI) has been used now as a research tool to predict the success rates of available treatment modalities such as ESWL, ureteroscopy, and PCNL. It has also been used to predict the passage of stones based on sizes on CT scan and position of stone in kidney or ureter. The prediction accuracy has been around 88% and prediction of complications around 77%. ML based algorithms were used based on stone sizes on CT scan. They were able to predict stone composition in uric acid stone with sizes more than 5 mm in 100% of cases. While the prediction accuracy for non-uric acid stones was 75%. Kazemi and Mirroshandel used an ensemble model using serum calcium, uric acid levels and clinical parameters (diabetes, hypertension) symptoms such as pain, nausea and vomiting. They reported an accuracy of 97.1% for prediction of stone composition [6].

18.4 Conclusion

As we see a progress in laboratory and other technical fields in biochemistry, we make sure progress towards offering a better solution to the most challenging problem of renal stone management and its recurring complications.

References

1. Cloutier J, Villa L, Traxer O, Daudon M. Kidney stone analysis: "give me your stone, I will tell you who you are!". World J Urol. 2015;33(2):157–69.
2. Pak CYC, Kaplan R, Bone H, Townsend J, Waters O. A simple test for the diagnosis of absorptive, resorptive and renal hypercalciurias. N Engl J Med. 1975;292(10):497–500.
3. Gaurav G. Urinary biochemical profile in urolithiasis: a case control study from Tamil Nadu. Vellore: Christian Medical College; 2008. http://www.repository-tnmgrmu.ac.in/3463/
4. Albright F, Henneman P, Benedict PH, Forbes AP. Idiopathic hypercalciuria (a preliminary report). Proc R Soc Med. 1953;46(12):31–5.
5. Bargagli M, Moochhala S, Robertson WG, Gambaro G, Lombardi G, Unwin RJ, et al. Urinary metabolic profile and stone composition in kidney stone formers with and without heart disease. J Nephrol. 2022;35(3):851–7.
6. Hameed BMZ, Shah M, Naik N, Rai BP, Karimi H, Rice P, et al. The ascent of artificial intelligence in endourology: a systematic review over the last 2 decades. Curr Urol Rep. 2021;22(10):53.

PCNL: Future Directions

19

The Future of PCNL

Subodh R. Shivde

There have been many developments in the field of percutaneous renal surgery and stone treatment in general. Developments have been occurring in designing the instruments and accessories such as baskets, guide wires and devices for the prevention of retrograde migration of stones [1]. The newer materials for Amplatz sheath have been thinner and more patient-friendly such as the use of Hickman Peel Away catheter sheaths, allowing their use in paediatric patients [2]. The newer generation of nephroscopes is getting slimmer ranging from mini to micro, rendering reduced complication rates without compromising efficiency [3].

Newer techniques used in laboratories include the coating of stones with ferromagnetic particles, thereby rendering them amenable to extraction with magnetic devices. Computer-developed models show good correlation with experimental results and appear to be a promising technology to improve stone-free status [4].

Increasing the use of novel scoring systems such as S.T.O.N.E. nephrometry would lead to better predictions of stone-free status and expected complications and morbidity [5]. Methods of grading patients with scores such as GUY'S stone score would help improve patient outcomes and help surgeons get realistic expectations out of the surgical exercise [6]. Machine learning based software would be used increasingly at institutions, as it compares very well to the established scores such as STONE morphometry and GUY'S stone score and shows better results in predicting outcomes [7].

S. R. Shivde (✉)
Department of Urology Transplant and Robotics, Deenanath Mangeshkar Hospital, Pune, India

S. R. Shivde (ed.), *Techniques in Percutaneous Renal Stone Surgery*, https://doi.org/10.1007/978-981-19-9418-0_19

Fluid extravasation and complications following PCNL are difficult to diagnose and manage subsequently, mainly due to the prone position in the majority of the patients. Ensuing compression caused due to fluid entrapment has been reported to cause rare complications such as abdominal compartment syndrome [8]. Other known complications during the PCNL surgery are the effects due to fluid or air in the pleural cavity such as hydrothorax or hemopneumothorax. Early use of ultrasound devices such as E Fast has been shown to be effective in identifying these life-threatening complications in the operation theatre itself and help insertion of drains to alleviate pressure-related situations even in the prone position [9].

Day care PCNL is being reported with increasing numbers [10]. PCNL as a modality is being tried with multiple tracks for larger stone volumes and even staghorn calculi. The reported series with total of 86 cases defined day care as admission for less than 24 h and have used both tubeless and use of nephrostomy tubes for a variable duration of up to 48 h. In the series by Wu et al. stone clearance was seen in 90.7% cases. The tract size ranged between 16 and 22 Fr. 60.5% cases were done by tubeless method. The reported complication rate was 11.6% with a re-admission rate 2.3%. The mean drop of Hb was 15.7 ± 16.9 g/L. It appears that the gap between aspirations and the reality of the day care PCNL is slowly narrowing [11].

Newer applications such as Stent Tracker tools are being evaluated and incorporated into the patient management systems leading to reduced incidence of 'Forgotten JJ Stent' entity. These simple and easy to use interfaces would eventually lead to reduced forgotten stents and the associated morbidity. This would go a long way in establishing patient safety [12].

There are reports of use of specially designed smartphone and tablet apps for the 3D reconstruction of the complex stone cases [13]. A recent small study by Vilares da Costa et al. demonstrated that such tools with the reconstruction of the CT images would help plan appropriate access in complex stone scenarios avoiding the access related vascular complications thereby enhancing patient safety.

A recent paper by Rassweiller et al. showed the use of iPad (Apple Inc. Cupertino) for kidney access. The authors used a matched pair group comparison to study PCNL using the said app and conventional approach with X-ray and USG to gain access to pelvicalyceal system. They found that there was a significant difference as regards exposure to X-ray, i.e. radiation and puncture time favouring conventional approach (p value < 0.01), and (p = 0.01) but the puncture attempts were the same in both groups (p value 0.45) [14].

Mobasheri et al. systematically reviewed 39 studies involving use of smartphones and tablets studied four major databases such as Embase, MEDLINE, Health Management Informatics and PsychINFO databases [15]. The studies had use of smartphones in 24 and tablets in 15. 30 studies used app-based interventions. Multiple domains tackled involved diagnostics, telemedicine, operative navigation, operative planning and patient education [14]. As more and more web-based and app-based applications keep coming out for the use of physicians and patients there would be an increasing need for monitoring these for quality, usability, ratings as regards data and user privacy. There would also be an urgent need for setting up regulatory controls and certifications. While certain programs such as Haptic Health App Certification program (HHAC)—a voluntary certification program, captures many features needed by an 'Ideal App' these remain restricted to a certain domain both geographical and speciality specific [16].

CT scan-guided access to pelvicalyceal system is reported to be close to 100%. 3D reconstruction allows a virtually complication free route to percutaneous access. Newer introductions to the urologist armamentarium include systems such as Uro Dyna CT (Siemens Healthcare Germany) [17]. It is an integration of conventional X-ray, fluoroscopy and 3D imaging. It also consists of a fully mobile carbon table with wireless control and allows cross-sectional reconstruction. The design allows user to do 3D planning with a laser-guided puncture tool.

While no field advancement would be complete without advances in the teaching and training, percutaneous renal surgery has not been an exception. Typically training for this type of surgery progresses from bench model to wet lab with the use of animal tissue or some organic matter [18] and then to virtual models. An objective assessment needs to be done with a surgical mentor to record enhanced proficiency before moving on to the modular operation theatre set up [19]. Rawandale et al. have developed a low cost, X-ray free PCNL simulator with the use of light and shadow as a simulator for X-ray image. It is simple to use, stress free and devoid of the use of computers making the learning of a complex task fairly easy and enjoyable [20].

The development of urologic technology started with transatlantic telesurgery by Prof. Rovetta in 1995, with a prostatic biopsy procedure. This was followed by telerobotics for the percutaneous puncture with the PAKY RCM Robot in 1996 [21]. These methods and the new tracker method allow precise puncture and safe beginning of a commonly done procedure such as PCNL. This method will find further applications such as biopsy of renal and tissue masses with tele-mentoring.

The modern urology practice is seeing use of 3D printing technology to produce models of kidney and stones using CT scan data. We are seeing the use in enhancing stone-free rates [22]. This new application is also finding its use in training the urology residents, making them understand the 3-dimensional anatomy and complexity of the stone volume. The same goes for use of these models to counsel patients and make them understand the complexity of operative procedure and help them choose the most appropriate procedure [23].

With the help of ever evolving technology and clinical expertise, we hope to move towards the elusive goal of 'zero complications' and 100% stone-free state after percutaneous renal stone surgery.

References

1. Rane A, Bradoo A, Rao P, Shivde S, Elhilali M, Anidjar M, Pace K, John RD. The use of a novel reverse thermosensitive polymer to prevent ureteral stone retropulsion during intracorporeal lithotripsy: a randomized, controlled trial. J Urol. 2010;183:1417–21. https://doi.org/10.1016/j.juro.2009.12.023.
2. Helal M, Black T, Lockhart J, Figueroa TE. The Hickman peel-away sheath: alternative for pediatric percutaneous nephrolithotomy. J Endourol. 1997;11:171–2. https://doi.org/10.1089/end.1997.11.171.
3. Lahme S. Miniaturisation of PCNL. Urolithiasis. 2018;46:99–106. https://doi.org/10.1007/s00240-017-1029-3.
4. Fernandez R, Tan YK, Kaberle W, Best SL, Olweny EO, Pearle MS, Gnade BE, McElroy SL, Cadeddu JA. Determining a performance envelope for capture of kidney stones functionalized with superparamagnetic microparticles. J Endourol. 2012;26:1227–30. https://doi.org/10.1089/end.2011.0598.
5. Okhunov Z, Friedlander JI, George AK, Duty BD, Moreira DM, Srinivasan AK, Hillelsohn J, Smith AD, Okeke Z. S.T.O.N.E. nephrolithometry: novel surgical classification system for kidney calculi. Urology. 2013;81:1154–60. https://doi.org/10.1016/j.urology.2012.10.083.
6. Thomas K, Smith NC, Hegarty N, Glass JM. The Guy's stone score—grading the complexity of percutaneous nephrolithotomy procedures. Urology. 2011;78:277–81. https://doi.org/10.1016/j.urology.2010.12.026.
7. Aminsharifi A, Irani D, Tayebi S, Jafari Kafash T, Shabanian T, Parsaei H. Predicting the postoperative outcome of percutaneous nephrolithotomy with machine learning system: software validation and comparative analysis with Guy's stone score and the CROES nomogram. J Endourol. 2020;34(6):692–9. https://doi.org/10.1089/end.2019.0475.
8. Tao J, Sheng L, Zhang H, Chen R, Sun Z-Q, Qian WQ. Acute abdominal compartment syndrome as a complication of percutaneous nephrolithotomy: two cases reports and literature review. Urol Case Rep. 2016;8:12–4. https://doi.org/10.1016/j.eucr.2016.05.001.
9. Sharma A, et al. eFAST for the diagnosis of a perioperative complication during percutaneous nephrolithotomy. Crit Ultrasound J. 2018;10:7. https://doi.org/10.1186/s13089-018-0088-1.
10. Wu X, Zhao Z, Sun H, Cai C, Li Z, Cheng D, Zhu H, Zeng G, Liu Y. Day-surgery percutaneous nephrolithotomy: a high-volume center retrospective experience. World J Urol. 2020;38:1323–8. https://doi.org/10.1007/s00345-019-02942-0.
11. Zhang S, Wu W, Huang YP, Wu W. Day-surgery percutaneous nephrolithotomy: a gap between inspiring results and the reality. World J Urol. 2020;38:1347–8. https://doi.org/10.1007/s00345-019-03006-z.
12. Molina WR, Pessoa R, da Silva D, Rodrigo K, McCabe C, Gustafson D, Nogueira L, Leo ME, Yu MK, Kim FJ. A new patient safety smartphone application for prevention of "forgotten" ureteral stents: results from a clinical pilot study in 194 patients. Patient Saf Surg. 2017;11:10. https://doi.org/10.1186/s13037-017-0123-3.
13. da Costa Vilares LA, Neto CLA, Dall'Aqua V, Covas MM, Machado MT, Menezes AD, Glina S. The role of interactive 3D reconstruction smartphone app on planning percutaneous nephrolithotomy surgery. J Urol. 2020;203:e333. https://doi.org/10.1097/JU.0000000000000855.014.
14. Rassweiler-Seyfried M-C, Rassweiler JJ, Weiss C, Müller M, Meinzer HP, Maier-Hein L, Klein JT. iPad-assisted percutaneous nephrolithotomy (PCNL): a matched pair analysis compared to standard PCNL. World J Urol. 2020;38:447–53. https://doi.org/10.1007/s00345-019-02801-y.
15. Mobasheri MH, Johnston M, Syed UM, King D, Darzi A. The uses of smartphones and tablet devices in surgery: a systematic review of the literature. Surgery. 2015;158:1352–71. https://doi.org/10.1016/j.surg.2015.03.029.

16. Boulos MN, Kamel B, Ann C, Karimkhani C, Buller DB, Dellavalle RP. Mobile medical and health apps: state of the art, concerns, regulatory control and certification. Online J Public Health Inform. 2014;5:229. https://doi.org/10.5210/ojphi.v5i3.4814.
17. Smith AD, Preminger G, Badlani GH, Kavoussi LR. Smith's textbook of endourology. New York: Wiley; 2019. https://books.google.co.in/books?id=nP2CDwAAQBAJ
18. Sinha M, Krishnamoorthy V. Use of a vegetable model as a training tool for PCNL puncture. Indian J Urol. 2015;31(2):156–9.
19. Aydın A, Al-Jabir A, Smith B, Ahmed K. Training in percutaneous nephrolithotomy. Singapore: Springer; 2020. https://doi.org/10.1007/978-981-15-0575-1_21.
20. Rawandale A, Patni L, Dar Y, GAutam Ladumor. PD19-03 construction and assessment of an innovative virtual (radiation free) fluoroscopy PCNL simulator: an indigenous approach to training. J Urol. 2016;195:e445–6. https://doi.org/10.1016/j.juro.2016.02.1402.
21. Challacombe BJ, Kavoussi LR, Dasgupta P. Trans-oceanic telerobotic surgery. BJU Int. 2003;92:678–80. https://doi.org/10.1046/j.1464-410X.2003.04475.x.
22. Xu Y, Yuan Y, Cai Y, Li X, Wan S, Xu G. Use 3D printing technology to enhance stone free rate in single tract percutaneous nephrolithotomy for the treatment of staghorn stones. Urolithiasis. 2019;48:509–16. https://doi.org/10.1007/s00240-019-01164-8.
23. Favorito LA. Kidney anatomy: three dimensional (3D) printed pelvicalyceal system models of the collector system improve the diagnosis and treatment of stone disease. Int Braz J Urol. 2017;43(3):381–2. https://www.scielo.br/scielo.php?script=sci_isoref&pid=S1677-55382017000300470&lng=en&tlng=en

GPSR Compliance

The European Union's (EU) General Product Safety Regulation (GPSR) is a set of rules that requires consumer products to be safe and our obligations to ensure this.

If you have any concerns about our products, you can contact us on ProductSafety@springernature.com

In case Publisher is established outside the EU, the EU authorized representative is:

Springer Nature Customer Service Center GmbH
Europaplatz 3
69115 Heidelberg, Germany

Batch number: 10370708

Printed by Printforce, the Netherlands